DIAGNOSTIC PROBLEMS IN TUMOR PATHOLOGY SERIES

DIAGNOSTIC PROBLEMS IN TUMORS OF HEAD AND NECK: SELECTED TOPICS

DIAGNOSTIC PROBLEMS IN TUMOR PATHOLOGY SERIES

Series Editors

Arun Chitale, MD (Path)

Diplomate American Board of Pathology (1969)
Surgical Pathologist
Sir HN Hospital, Jaslok Hospital, Surgical Pathology Center
Formerly Professor & Head Department of Pathology Bombay Hospital Institute of Medical Sciences, Mumbai, India

Dhananjay Chitale, MD (Path) DNB (Path)

Diplomate American Board of Pathology
Division Head, Molecular Pathology & Genomic Medicine,
Senior Staff Surgical Pathologist
Director, Tissue Biorepostiroy
Assistant Clinical Professor, Wayne State University School of Medicine
Henry Ford Hospital, Detroit, Michigan, USA

Diagnostic Problems in Tumors of Head and Neck: Selected Topics, 1/e
Arun Chitale, Dhananjay Chitale, 2014

Published by Arun Chitale & Dhananjay Chitale

DIAGNOSTIC PROBLEMS IN TUMORS OF HEAD AND NECK: SELECTED TOPICS

Authors

Arun Chitale, MD (Path)
Diplomate American Board of Pathology (1969)
Surgical Pathologist
Sir HN Hospital, Jaslok Hospital, Surgical Pathology Center
Formerly Professor & Head Department of Pathology Bombay Hospital Institute of Medical Sciences, Mumbai, India

Dhananjay Chitale, MD (Path) DNB (Path)
Diplomate American Board of Pathology
Division Head, Molecular Pathology & Genomic Medicine,
Senior Staff Surgical Pathologist
Director, Tissue Biorepostiroy
Assistant Clinical Professor, Wayne State University School of Medicine
Henry Ford Hospital, Detroit, Michigan, USA

Acknowledgements

Drs Ashok Mehta and Vijay Haribhakti, oncosurgeons in Mumbai have graciously contributed all clinical photographs of oral cancers: Figures- 2, 4 A&B, 6 A, 7 C, 9 C, 13 A&B, 16 & 17.
Figure 14 A-pseudoepitheliomatous hyperplasia or oral cavity contributed by Dr K G Naik, Pathologist, Surat
Figures 37A-K:PLGA, 38 F: Low grade salivary duct carcinoma mimicking cystadenoma, Figure 40A-H: Myoepithelial Carcinoma: Cases provided Courtesy: Dr. Richard J. Zarbo, Henry Ford Hospital, Detroit, Michigan, USA
Figure 46: A-D- Teratocarcinosarcoma & Figure 49 C- S 100 positive sustentacular cells in paraganglioma Courtesy Dr Anita Borges, Surgical Pathologist, Raheja Hospital, Mumbai

Table of Contents

PREFACE:

DIAGNOSTIC PROBLEMS IN SURGICAL PATHOLOGY:

Uncommon presentation of common lesions and rare lesions

Histopathological evaluation is the gold standard in the diagnosis of malignant tumors and chronic diseases of visceral organs like liver, kidney and lungs. Histopathological analysis provides information that helps the clinician to choose the most appropriate treatment modality and assists in prognostication. Notwithstanding the current and future advances in the imaging technology and other innovations, the status of Histopathology will remain unchanged for decades to come.

Whereas Histopathology is the most objective form of investigation, there are many gray areas in arriving at a definitive diagnosis. On many occasions total lack of clinical information leads to avoidable errors in the diagnosis. The surgical pathologist is advised to keep the cases pending until adequate information is available. On the other hand there are numerous problems in histological interpretation even if the entire clinical information is at hand. This occurs because some lesions have inherent morphological ambiguities and no two surgical pathologists may agree on the correct histological diagnosis. One such lesion, for example, is verrucous squamous cell carcinoma of the oro-pharyngeal region or other organs with squamous epithelial lining. The most controversial problem in thyroid disorders is a lesion called follicular variant of papillary carcinoma. In every organ and system, there are sporadic entities, which have debatable criteria of morphological diagnosis. The object of this book is to adequately address problems of uncommon morphologic variations of common lesions and rare difficult lesions with the help of extensive illustrations. There are excellent frequently updated textbooks of surgical pathology, in which all lesions occurring in various sites are described, illustrated and backed by references. However, due to constraints of space, these problematic entities are not extensively illustrated or explained at length. This deficiency is admirably handled in exclusively individual organ pathology monograms. However, this requires the facility of a well-stocked library; most practicing surgical pathologists do not have access to these.

The proposed book is an attempt to address these lesions with multiple illustrations and detailed pertinent text. It is envisaged that the book should be a companion to a standard surgical pathology textbook and this should be accessible just at the fingertips via power of electronic media using internet. The targeted audience includes residents in Anatomic Pathology; young recently qualified pathologists and a large contingent of pathologists attached to medical institutions, in which the volume of surgical specimens is low.

Note on statistical data presented in this eBook:

The senior author (ARC) has been a practicing consultant surgical pathologist for the last 44 years (1969-2013). As a surgical pathologist, he has been associated with 'surgical pathology center' (his own lab). He is also attached to the following hospitals in Mumbai (Bombay): Sir H N Hospital, Bombay Hospital and Jaslok Hospital (all corporate institutions), Bone Registry, Grant Medical College; Cytology department of KEM Hospital.

He has gathered vast amount of neoplastic cases of different organ-systems and the data has been in the form of Tables for different organ systems. The statistical tabulation of tumors has been based on classification of anatomical site and behavior (benign or malignant). This is not purported to be a population based epidemiological data. However, the data likely represents a fair cross sectional distribution and representation of various neoplasms in the population served in Metropolitan Mumbai (Bombay), India.

DISCLAIMER:

This Book titled Diagnostic Problems in Tumors of Head and Neck: Selected Topics, is made available by the Authors solely for trained and licensed physician for personal, non-commercial teaching and educational use. No two individual patients with neoplasms are identical and therefore diagnosis and treatment varies greatly depending on the medical and surgical history. The information contained in this Book is not medical advice. It is the professional responsibility of the practitioner to apply the information provided in a specific situation. Attention has been taken for accuracy of the information presented to describe generally accepted practices; however, knowledge and best practice in the field constantly change with new research. Readers are advised to check the most current information. The authors, editors and publishers are not responsible for errors or omissions or for any outcomes from the use of the information in this book and make no warranty, expressed or implied, with respect to the currency, completeness or accuracy of the content of the publication. This educational application is not a medical device and does not and should not be construed to provide health related or medical advice, or clinical decision support or to support or replace the diagnosis, recommendation, advise, treatment or decision by an appropriately trained licensed physician, including, without limitation with respect to any life sustaining or lifesaving treatment or decision. This educational material does not create a physician patient relationship between the authors and any individual. Before making any medical or health related decision, individuals, including those with any neoplasms are advised to consult an appropriately trained and licensed physician. To the fullest extent of the law, the authors, the editors or the publisher do not assume any liability for any injury and/or damage to persons or property arising out of or related to any use of the material contained in this book.

Squamous Cell Carcinoma of Upper Aero-digestive Tract

Introduction:

Eggston & Woff published the first ever book of "Histopathology of the Ear, Nose and Throat" in 1947. The first two of the initial series of atlases published by Armed Forces Institute of Pathology (AFIP) included Salivary Gland Tumors by Foote & Frazell in1954 and An Atlas of Otolaryngic Pathology by Ash & Raum in 1956. John Bastakis (pathologist from M D Anderson Centre) wrote a book on 'Tumors of Head and Neck', which was published in 1974. This marked a major event in the emergence of Head & Neck pathology into a fully mature discipline. In the field of oncology, Head and Neck surgery is a well-established and an important medical subspecialty.

The various anatomical regions included under the rubric Head & Neck are: upper aero-digestive tract, nose and paranasal sinuses, salivary glands, ear, eye and orbit. A total of 19665 biopsies and resected specimens from these sites have been signed out by the author in a 40 year period (1970 to 2010, Table I). Squamous cell carcinoma of upper aero-digestive tract constitutes a single most prevalent lesion in the Head and Neck. It is estimated that over 500,000 patients are diagnosed with cancer in this anatomical region the world over (WHO, 2005). Squamous cell carcinomas constitute 83% of total 7249 specimens from the aero digestive tract in our experience (Table 1).

Table 1: Site-wise biopsy specimens of head and neck (n=19665) Author's Series 1970-2005	
Oral Cavity and Oropharynx	6821 (34.70%)
Epiglottis, Supraglottic larynx & vocal cords	5478 (27.85%)
Sino nasal tract	2855 (14.51%)
Major salivary glands	1679 (08.53%)
Jaws	1172 (05.95%)
Nasopharynx	0480 (02.44%)
Ear	0764 (03.88%)
Eye & Orbit	0416 (02.11%)

Table 2: Squamous Carcinoma of Aero-digestive Tract: Site-wise (total n=5487). Author's series 1970			
Anterior Tongue	947	Posterior pharynx	65
Cheek	669	Floor of Mouth	32
Hypopharynx	566	Angle of Mouth	27
Tonsil	307	Upper lip	14
Posterior Tongue	223	Nasopharynx	206
Gums	217	Epiglottis	119
Lower lip	156	Supraglottic	1343
Palate	106	Vocal Cord	482

Almost 65% (3525/5487) of squamous cell carcinomas of aero-digestive tract occurred in anterior tongue, cheek, hypopharynx and supraglottic larynx (Table 2). Oral cancer is a serious disease which in many cases has a disastrous outcome. Cancer and its sequelae may cause heavy impairment in life quality and it is associated with suffering for patients, as well as for their relatives and friends. Despite easy accessibility of the oral cavity to direct examination, this cancer is often not detected until at a late stage. As a result, the survival rate for oral cancer has remained essentially unchanged over the past 3 decades.

It is well established that most oral carcinomas develop from premalignant lesions, which cause noticeable clinical and histological changes in the oral mucosa. Detection of precursor or premalignant lesions is thus of the highest priority in an attempt to prevent occurrence of invasive squamous carcinoma. It has been reported that 15% of asymptomatic oral lesions were larger than 4 cm at the initial presentation. Surgical pathologist has an important role to play, which involves accurate histological diagnosis of these lesions. Squamous cell carcinoma of oral cavity is often under or over diagnosed. There are many proliferative lesions with some overlap and variable rate of malignant transformation. Diagnostic difficulties particularly in the grading of dysplasia and identification of verrucuous squamous cell carcinoma require special attention and care (1, 2, 3 , 4.)

Epithelial Precursor ("Precancerous") Lesions:

Oral precancerous lesions include leukoplakia, erythroplakia, lichen planus and submucous fibrosis. These lesions are clinically recognized premalignant lesions and transformation to invasive carcinoma occurs after a widely variable interval. These usually asymptomatic mucosal alterations are biopsied in order to assess the presence of dysplasia and to know its grade. In some cases, a clinically inapparent invasive squamous carcinoma has been detected beneath or in the vicinity of a leukoplakic patch (Table 3).

Table 3: Epithelial Precursor (Premalignant) Lesions** of Aero-digestive Tract (n = 802) Author's series(1970-2005)	
Leukoplakia	564 (70.32)
Erythroplakia	106 (13.21)
Lichen Planus	82 (10.22)
Submucous Fibrosis	50 (06.23)

*Papilloma (total 412 cases) of the upper aero-digestive tract are not included because of rather low or even debatable malignant potential.

Leukoplakia

This has been defined (WHO) as a white or gray patch or plaque that cannot be removed or scraped. Clinically, leukoplakia may be of homogeneous type and appears flat, thin and uniformly white in color. The estimated prevalence of oral leukoplakia, worldwide, is reported to be over a wide range due to different geographic population distribution, age, gender, and clinical variability in diagnostic criteria. Overall, the prevalence is approximately 2 percent and the extent of its precancerous role has been controversial. Most of the initial studies on the subject showed a risk of malignant transformation in the range of 3 to 6 percent. Petti's reported (2003) pooled estimate of world leukoplakia prevalence from metaanalysis is 1.49%-2.60%). Using this data, he reported crude annual oral cancer incidence rate attributable to leukoplakia between 6.2 and 29.1 per 100,000, thus suggesting that the global number of oral cancer cases is probably underreported (5a). However, several more recent studies have shown more alarming malignant transformation rates ranging from 8.9 to 17.5 per cent (5, 5a, 6 & 7).

Histologically, a leukoplakic patch shows moderate to marked keratosis on the surface and thick acanthotic squamous epithelium (Figure 1 a-d). Minimal chronic inflammation may be seen in the immediate submucosal layer in some cases. Majority of the cases show no nuclear atypia but a fair number display dysplasia. (Figure 1) It cannot be too strongly emphasized that clinically diagnosed leukoplakia may histologically show a wide range of phenotypes such as hyperkeratosis, dysplasia or even invasive carcinoma (Figure.2). It is evident that a white patch in any part of oral mucosa should be taken seriously and promptly biopsied to look for dysplasia or clinically in-apparent underlying invasive carcinoma.

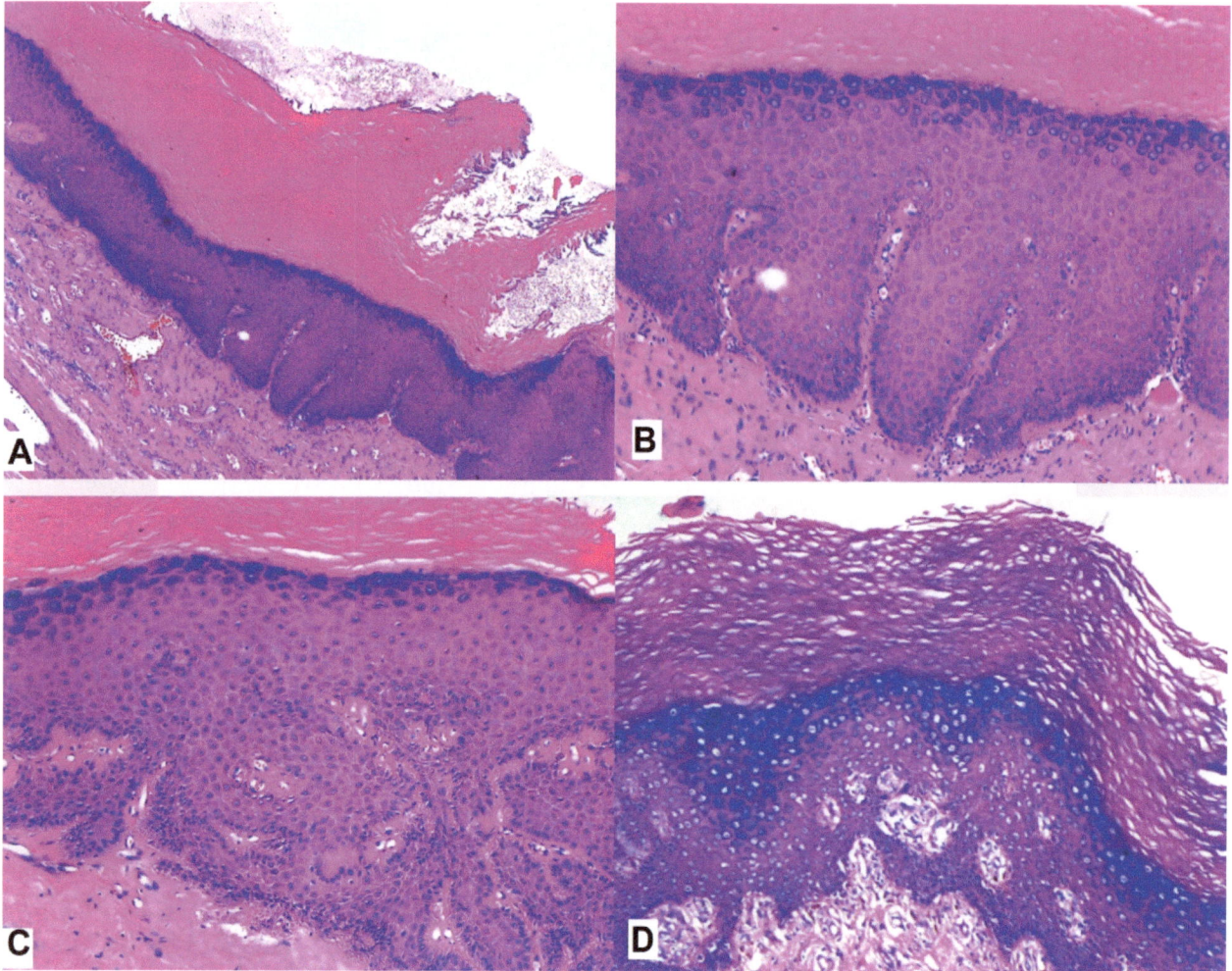

Figure 1A-D Leukoplakia: marked keratosis (orthokeratin) and mild mucosal thickening (A), a significant acanthotic thickening of squamous mucosa without dysplasia (B & C), broad layer of parakeratosis prominent granular cell layer and acanthosis (D)

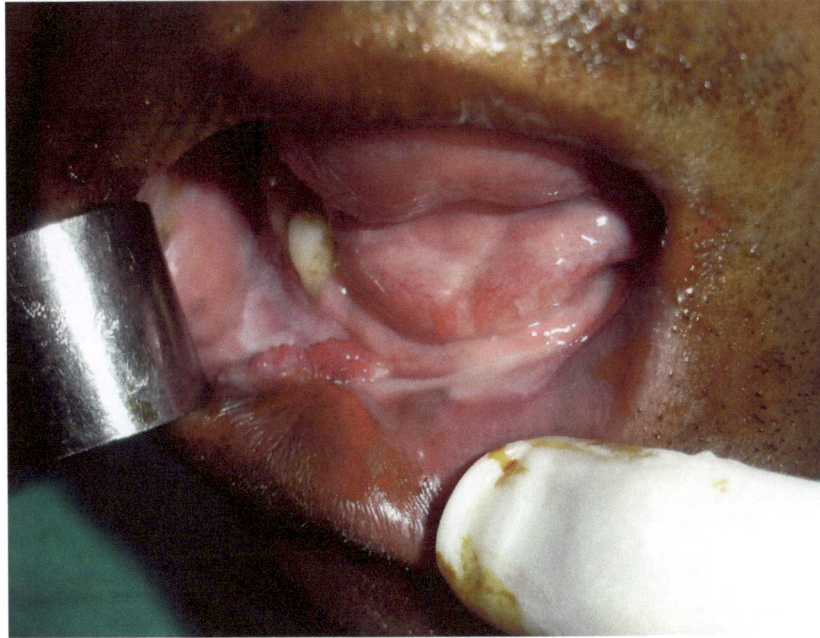

Figure 2 Leukoplakia and adjacent reddish granular growth in gingivo-buccal sulcus

Erythroplakia

Erythroplakia is defined in a similar way as Leukoplakia, being a fiery red patch that cannot be removed. Erythroplakia and its variant speckled leukoplakia harbor moderate to marked degree of dysplasia (Figure 3 A-D). The speckled leukoplakia is intermediate between leukoplakia and erythroplakia. The redness in these mucosal lesions is attributed to presence of significant dysplasia (Figure 4 A to D) The new WHO classification recognized that problem exists with the subjective nature of assessment of dysplasia and variation in its grading.

The grading system for intraepithelial neoplasia has been well established for uterine cervix. It is reproducible and many pathologists tend to extrapolate it to epithelial precursor lesions in the oral cavity. However, the classical non-keratinized type of carcinoma in situ of cervix (Figure 4 e & f) is rarely encountered in oral lesions. In fact, most of the intraepithelial neoplasms in upper aero-digestive tract are keratinizing type of dysplasias (Figure 3 A-D). The risk of developing invasive squamous carcinoma in mild, moderate and severe dysplasia is reported to be 5.7, 22.5 and 28.4% respectively. It is difficult to precisely define the grades of dysplasia, particularly moderate dysplasia. There is significant difference in inter-observer and intra-observer interpretation on the same case seen by different experienced pathologists (8).

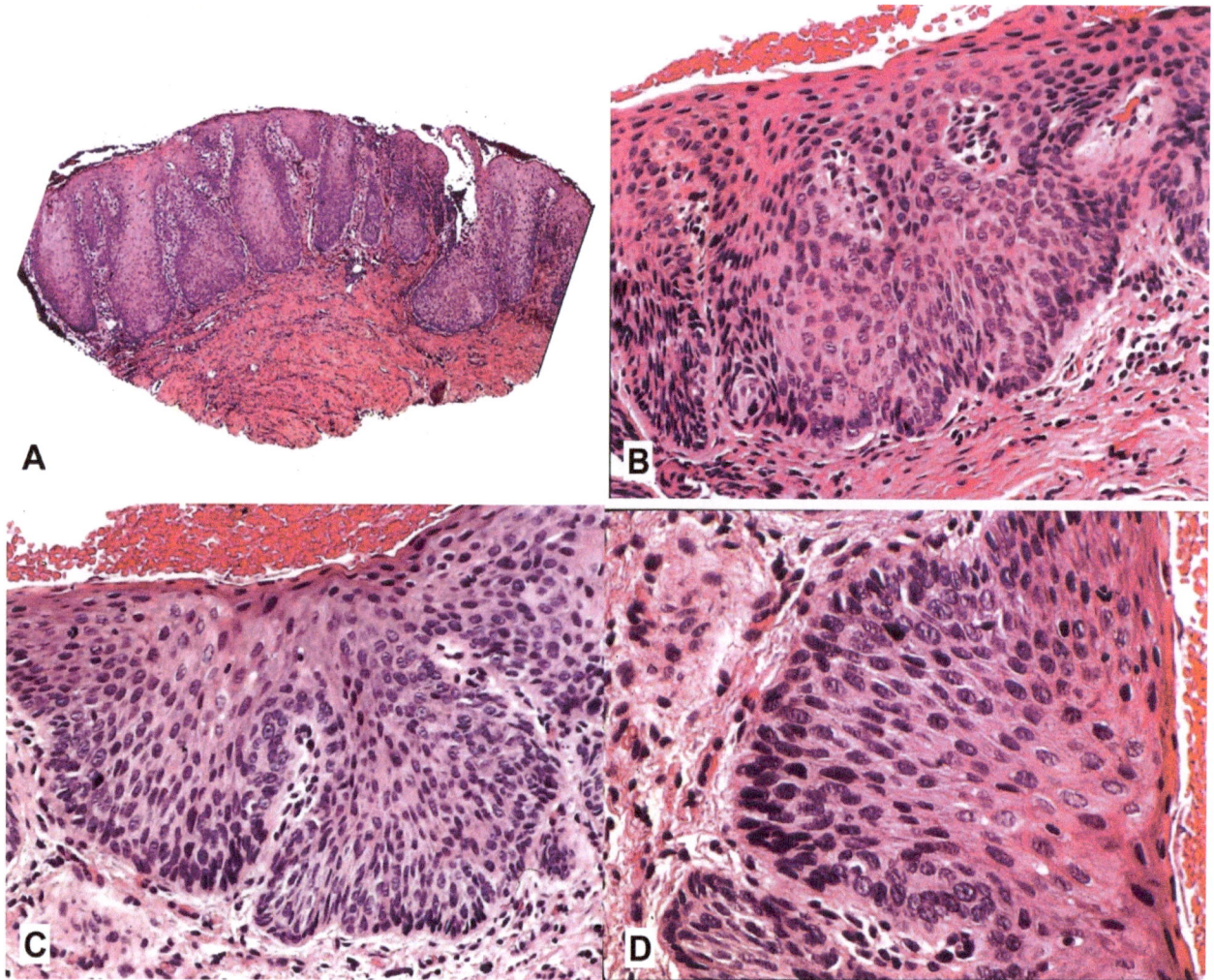

Figure 3 A-D Clinically Erythroplakia: Acanthosis with moderate dysplasia

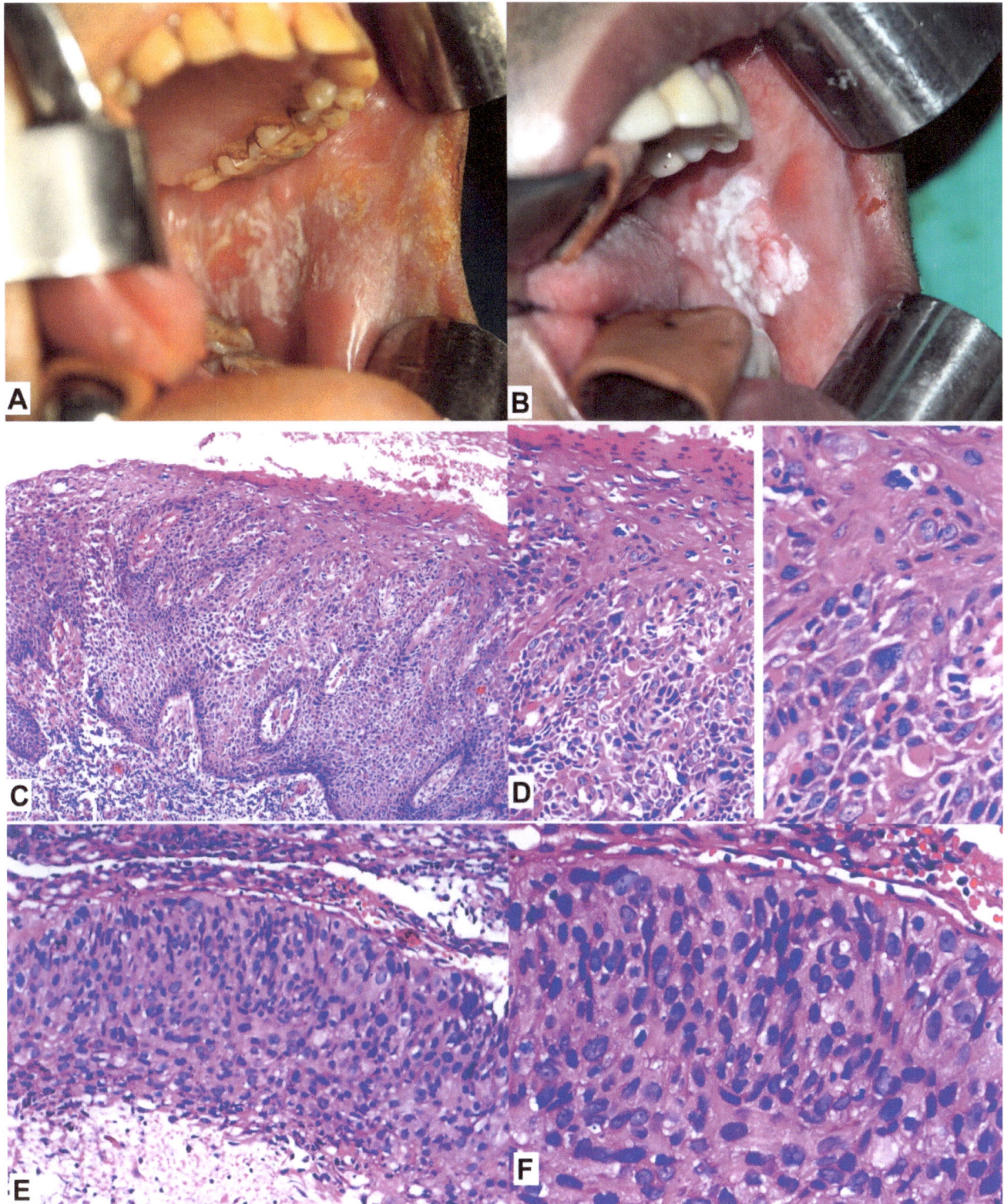

Figure 4 Severe dysplasia/CIS: a reddish plaque (erythroplakia): (A) red plaque and (B) partly white plaque, severe dysplasia of keratinized type (C&D) in buccal cavity of this case, (E & F) CIS of non keratinized type in the cervix for comparison

Table 4: Risk Factors of Significance for Malignant transformation of leukoplakia
Female gender
Leukoplakia in non-smokers
Long duration of leukoplakia
Non-homogenous patch
Location on tongue or floor of mouth
Size = >4 cm
Presence of dysplasia
DNA aneuploidy

Verrucous hyperplasia

Histologically, verrucous hyperplasia and carcinoma will have identical surface verrucous projections but verrucous proliferation does not extend as deep into underlying stroma as verrucous carcinoma does (Figure 5 A-B).

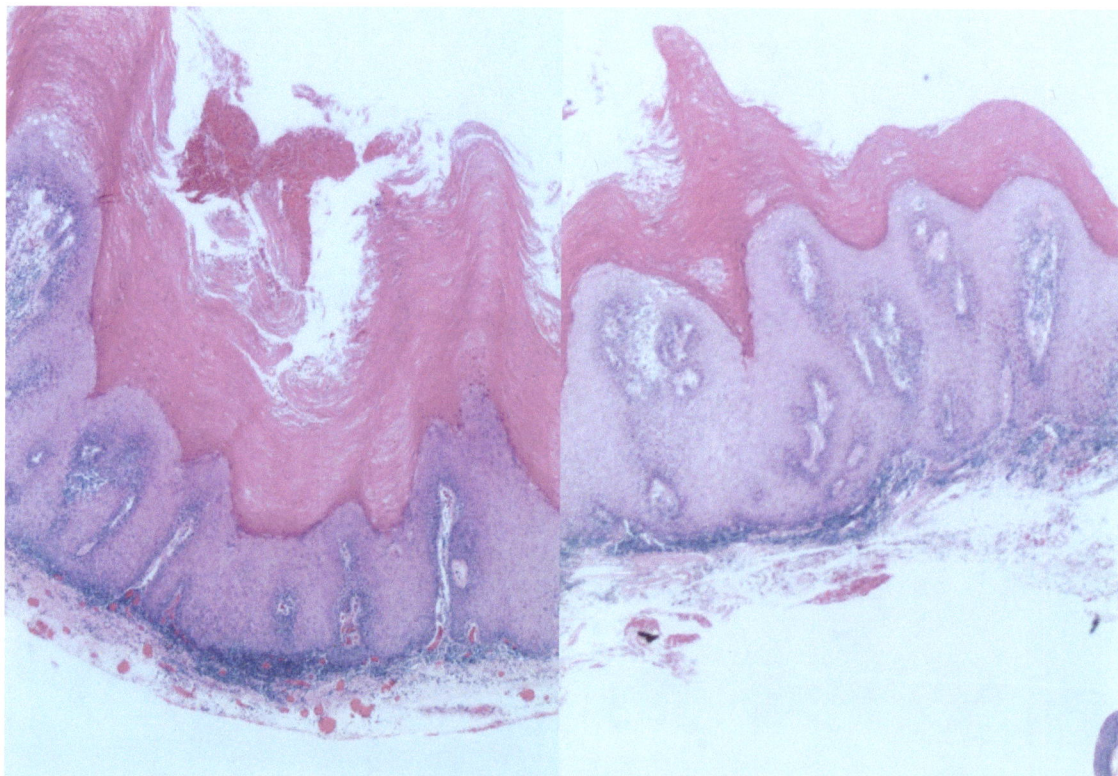

Figure 5 Verrucous hyperplasia: (A&B) acanthotic and papillomatous squamous proliferation with prominent keratosis, the base of the lesion is sharply delineated

Verrucous leukoplakia

The condition begins with conventional flat white patch that, over time tends to become much thicker and uneven in nature (Figure 6 a). Leukoplakia after some years progressively develops dysplastic changes (Figure 6 B, C)

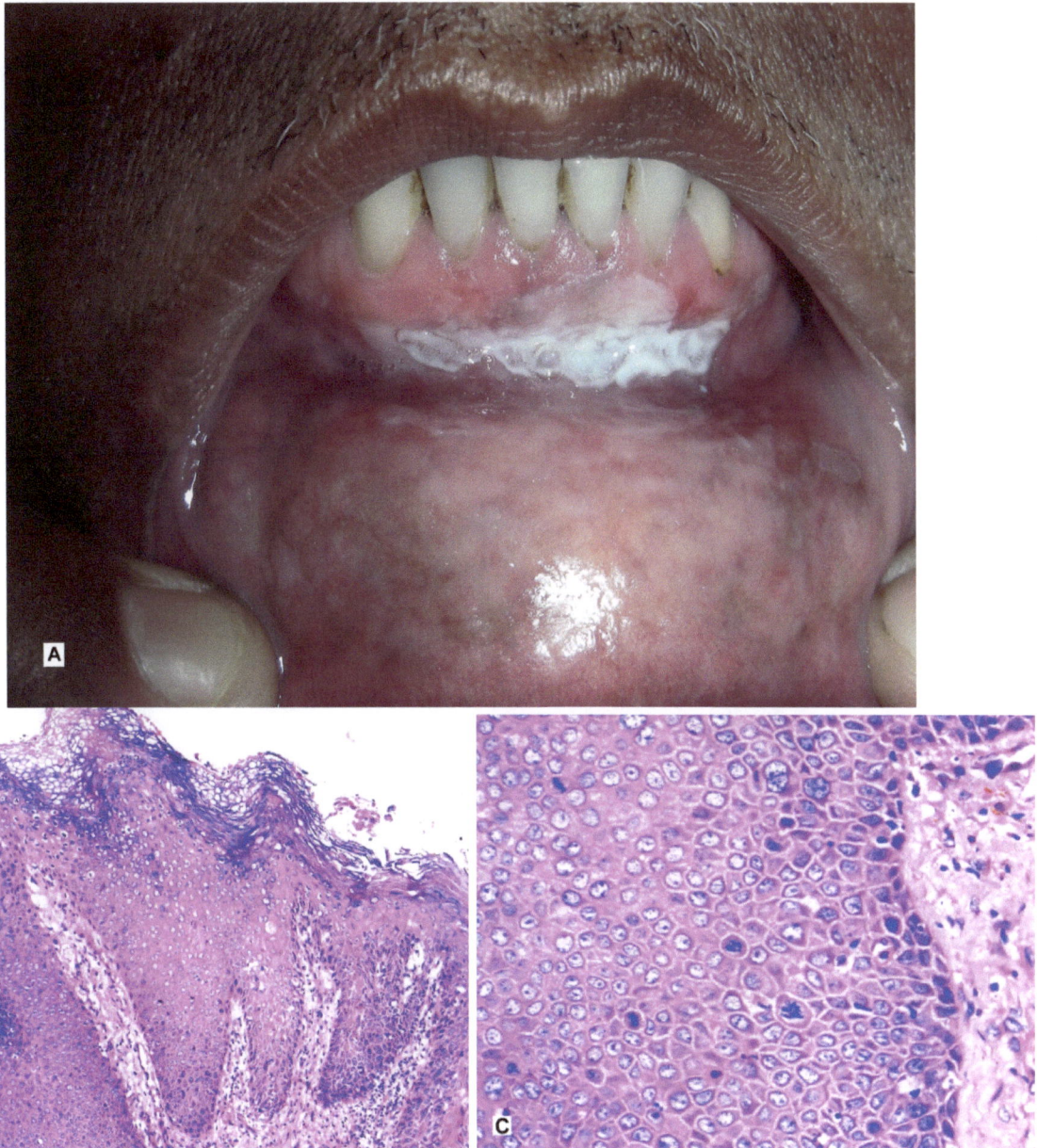

Figure 6 (A-C) A case of verrucous Leukoplakia of gums. A) Verrucous leukoplakia of gums; (B) keratoparakeratosis, papillomatosis and acanthosis; (C) mild to moderate dysplasia

A particularly aggressive type of leukoplakia, known as proliferative verrucous leukoplakia (Figure 7 A-B), is characterized by widespread, multifocal sites of involvement often in patients without known risk factors and more frequent in women (ratio of F:M =4:1). It progresses from hyperkeratosis to verrucuous hyperplasia to verrucous or conventional squamous cell carcinoma (Figure 7 C).

Proliferative verrucous leukoplakia and verrucous hyperplasia represent interrelated and irreversible mucosal lesions of the upper aero-digestive tract.

These verrucous lesions, according to some, represent an early biological form of verrucous carcinoma. The authors believe this proposition and when in difficulty we call the initial lesion atypical verrucous hyperplasia with a recommendation that wide local excision may have curative role (9).

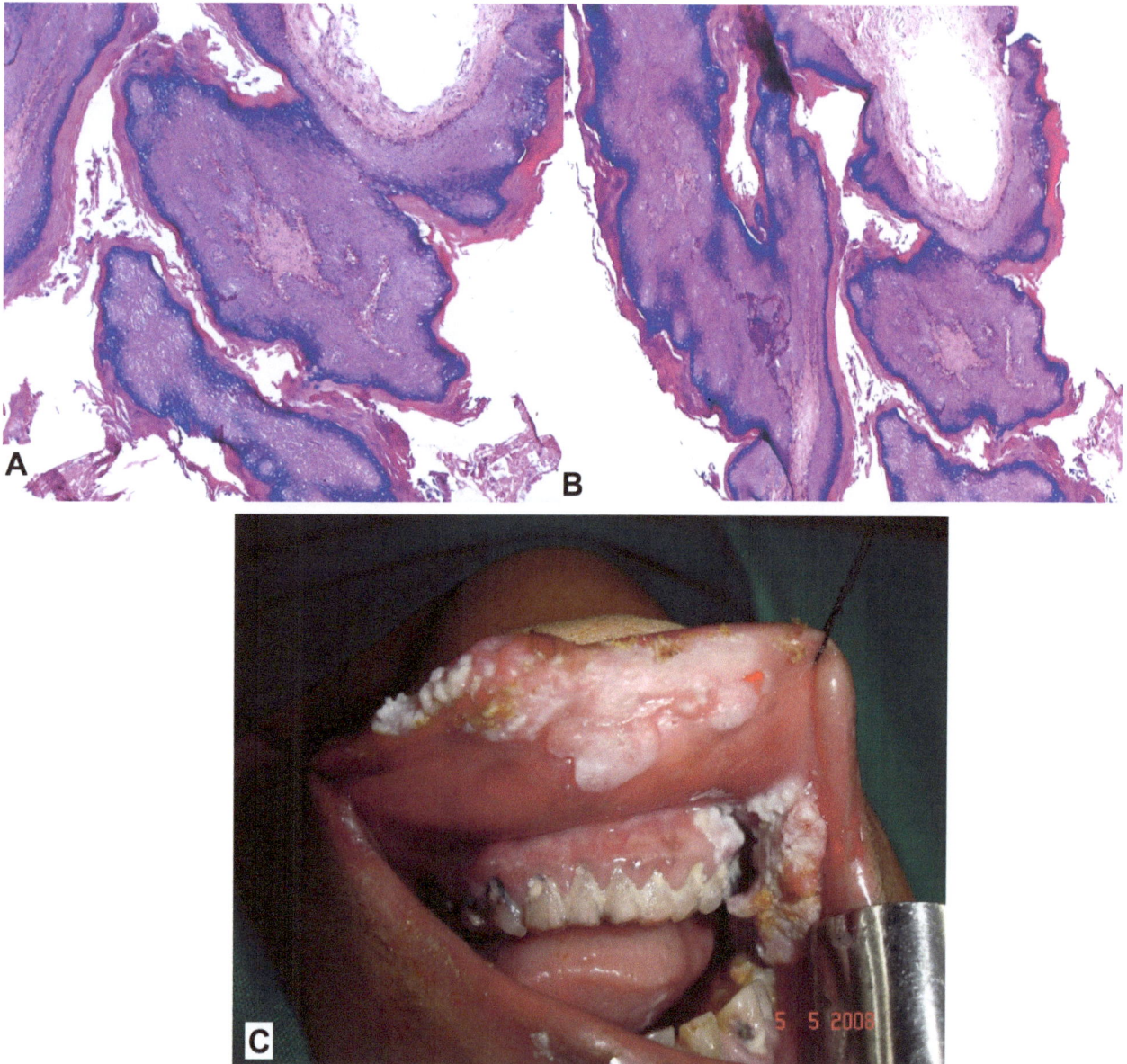

Figure 7 (A-C) Proliferative verrucous leukoplakia with two independent lesions (A&B), patient developed bicentric invasive squamous cell carcinoma 14 months after the first biopsy (C)

Lichen Planus

Oral lichen planus is a chronic muco-cutaneous immune inflammatory condition and occurs in 0.5 to 2.2 percent population with a peak incidence in the third to sixth decade. Its precancerous role is debatable or controversial. There has not been enough data to predict malignant transformation of lichen planus. However, it has been proposed that lichenoid oral lesion accompanied by dysplasia may progress to squamous carcinoma and that epithelial dysplasia with lichenoid features is a distinct histopathological entity with a true malignant predisposition. The morphological features of lichen planus include hyperkeratosis and irregular acanthosis with a prominent band of inflammation at the base with dissolution of basal layer (Figure 8 A-D). Lichenoid dysplasia designates the histological combination of mucosal epithelial dysplasia and few features of lichen planus, mainly pattern of inflammatory infiltrate. It has been shown that in oral lichen planus, cell proliferation rate was found to be less than in oral epithelial dysplasia and squamous carcinoma (10, 11, 12).

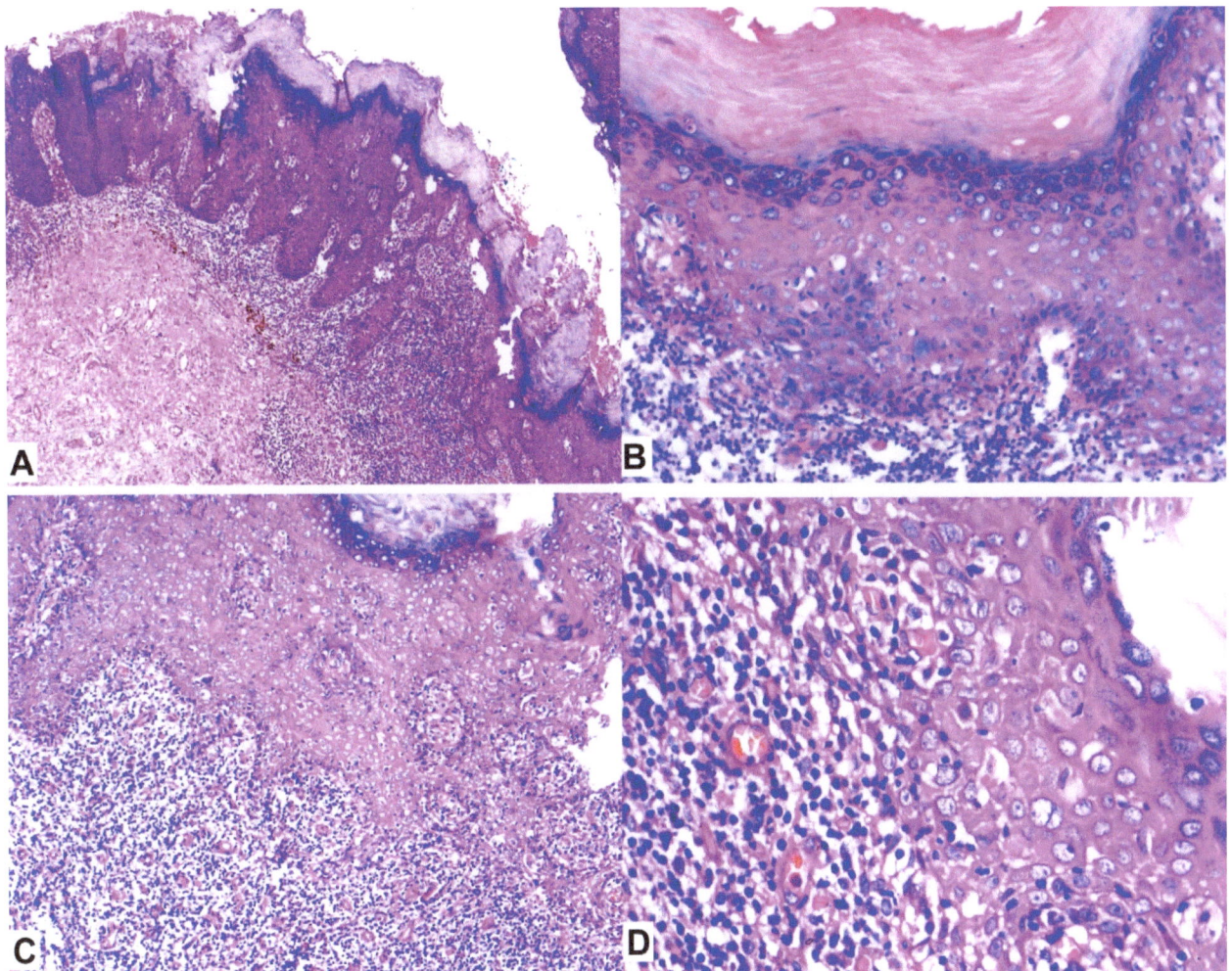

Figure 8 Oral Lichen Planus: (A, B), keratosis, acanthosis, prominent granular cell layer and band of chronic inflammation at the base note patchy loss of basal layer of the mucosa due to inflammatory destruction (C, D).

Submucous fibrosis

This is a chronic progressive condition of oral mucosa, in which clinically there is mucosal rigidity of varying intensity due to fibro elastic transformation of the juxtaepithelial connective tissue (Figure 9 A, B). It is associated with areca nut chewing, either alone or part of betel quid. Clinically it is characterized by burning sensation in the oral cavity, blanching, and stiffening of the oral and oropharyngeal region and leading to difficulty in opening the mouth (Figure 9 C). The symptoms and signs depend on the progression of the lesions and number of affected sites. It is predominantly seen in Indians and other Asians. Once the disease has developed, there is neither regression nor any effective treatment.

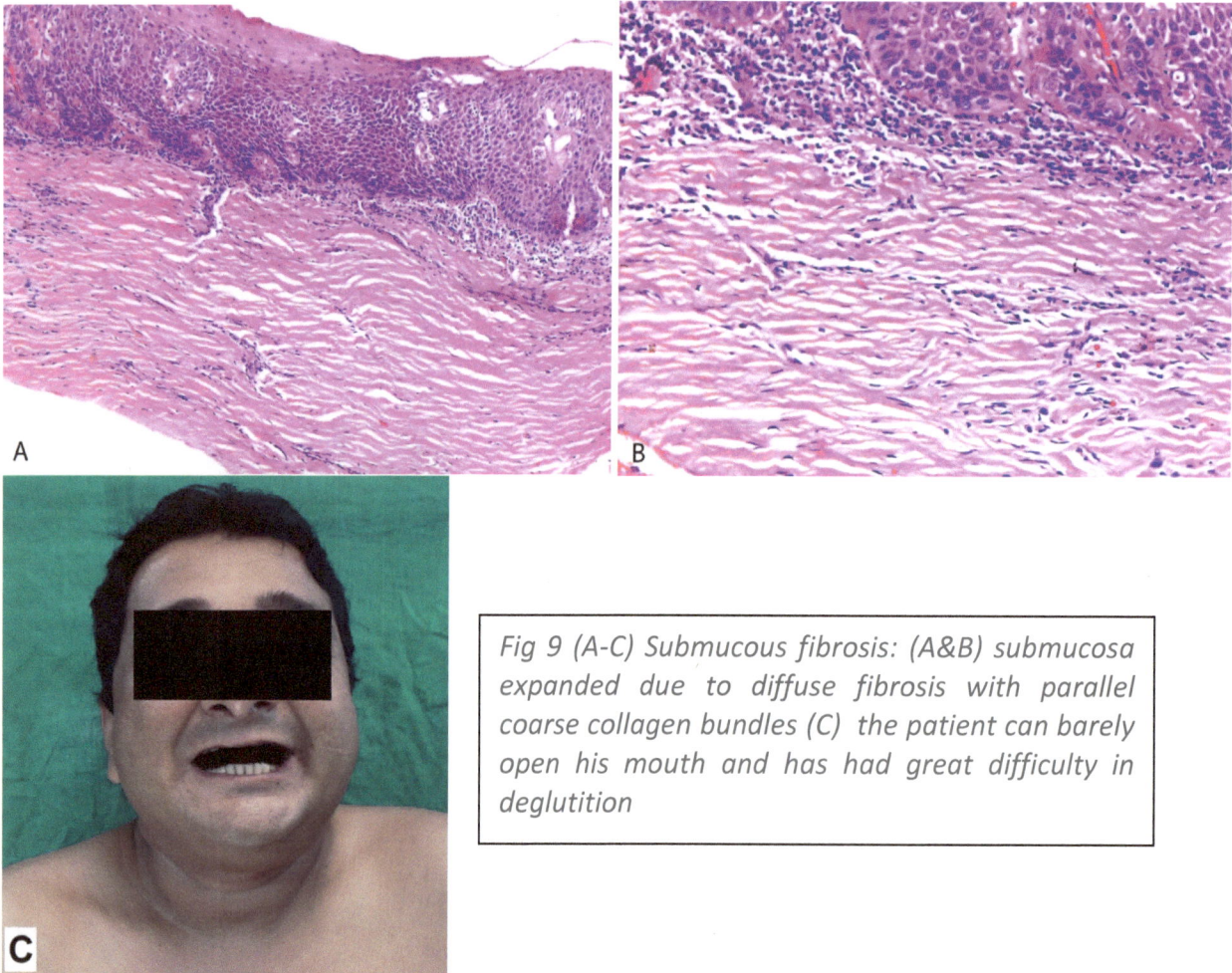

Fig 9 (A-C) Submucous fibrosis: (A&B) submucosa expanded due to diffuse fibrosis with parallel coarse collagen bundles (C) the patient can barely open his mouth and has had great difficulty in deglutition

The biopsy shows keratosis, mucosal atrophy and fibrosed submucosa. A variable degree of dysplasia is seen in up to 25% of cases.

One Indian population based study reported that squamous carcinoma developed in 7% of patients with submucous fibrosis, followed over a period of 17 years. In a recent review on the subject, nearly 12% of 205 patients developed carcinoma and this occurred predominantly in males (13).

Papilloma

The term papilloma of aero-digestive system is reserved for squamous mucosal proliferation with exophytic growth pattern characterized by a fibro-vascular core covered with keratotic thick acanthotic squamous epithelium (Figure 10 A & B). Squamous papilloma with atypia or dysplasia will rarely progress to CIS or invasive carcinoma. Isolated solitary papilloma is most common in the oral cavity, whereas multiple and recurring papillomas occur typically in larynx. In children, the laryngeal papillomas can recur over many years but display benign behavior. The recurrence can be large and may compromise the airway (Figure 11). Major clinical series' of juvenile onset papillomatosis rarely identify an occasional papilloma with malignant transformation, usually many years after onset of the disease. Dysplasia occurring in proliferating papillomatosis of the adolescent population is rarely a cause for concern. However, the same degree of dysplasia in adults with a papillary tumor is more complex and includes differential diagnosis of proliferative or recurrent papillomatosis, dysplastic papilloma, papillary carcinoma in situ or papillary carcinoma with or without invasion. An erroneous diagnosis of cancer in papillomatosis containing dysplasia is not uncommon. In general, biopsies from patients with recurrent papillomatosis should be evaluated with care. Malignancy in this small select group of cases should be based on demonstration of invasive squamous cell carcinoma.

Almost all recurrent papillomas of larynx are caused by HPV types 6 or 11 (Figure 12 A-C). It is interesting to know that these viruses have also been isolated from normal laryngeal mucosa of papilloma in remission.

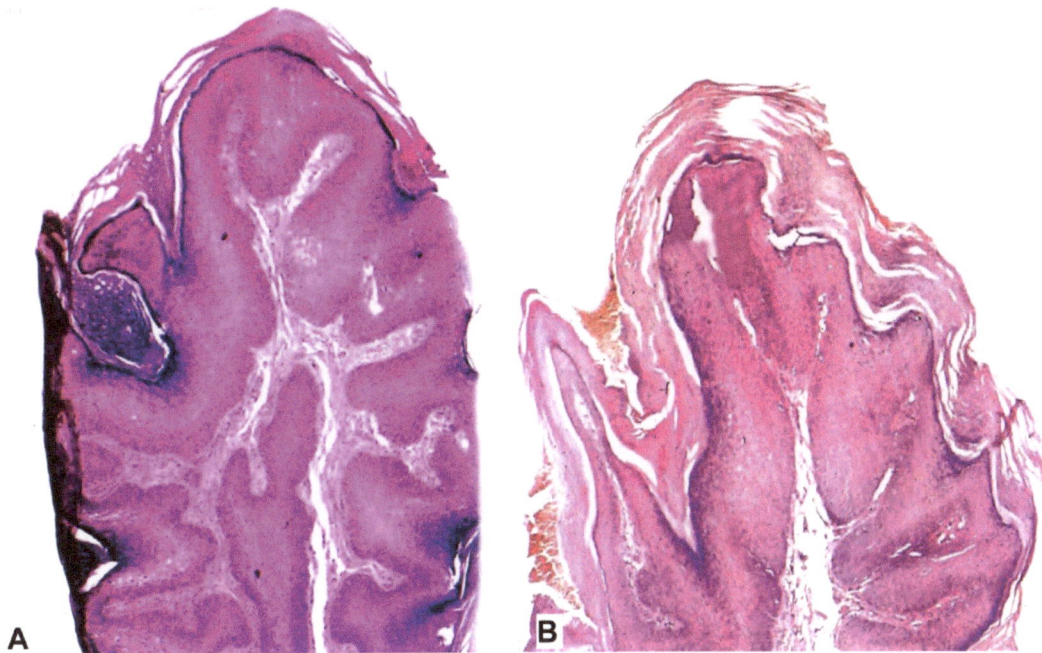

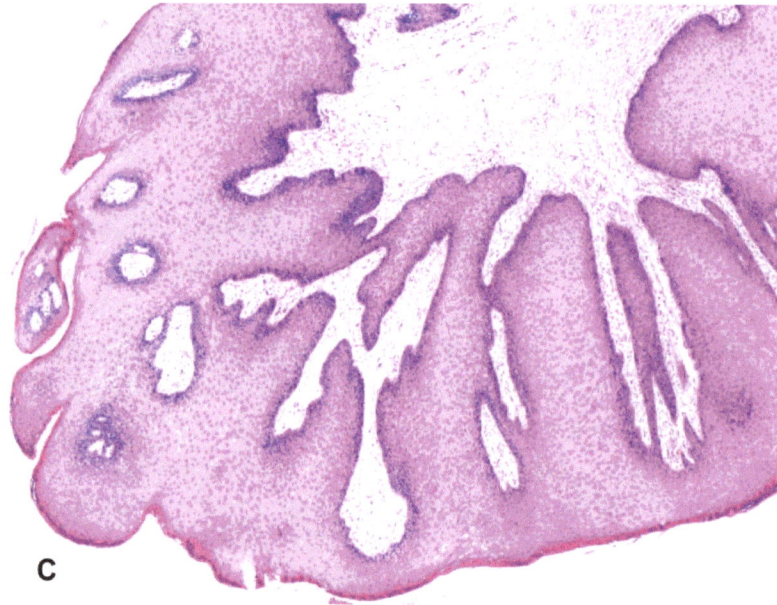

Figure 10 Papilloma: one from oral cavity (A) and other from epiglottis (B), both display central thin fibrous stalk and overlying keratotic acanthotic squamous mucosa. (C) Squamous papilloma of vocal cord.

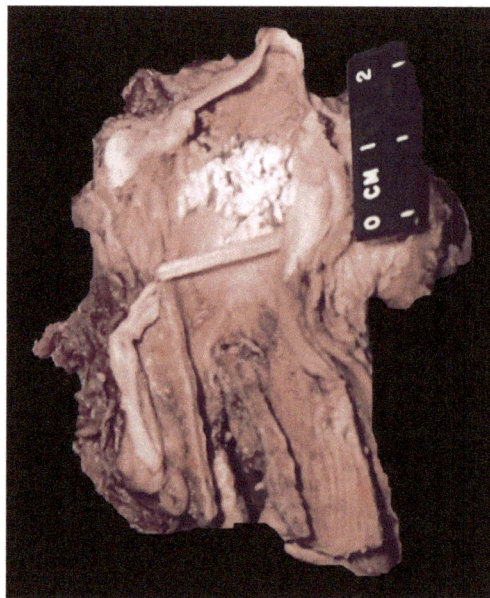

Figure 11 Larynx from a 35 year old patient, who succumbed to benign papillomatosis of the glottis, no malignant change was present

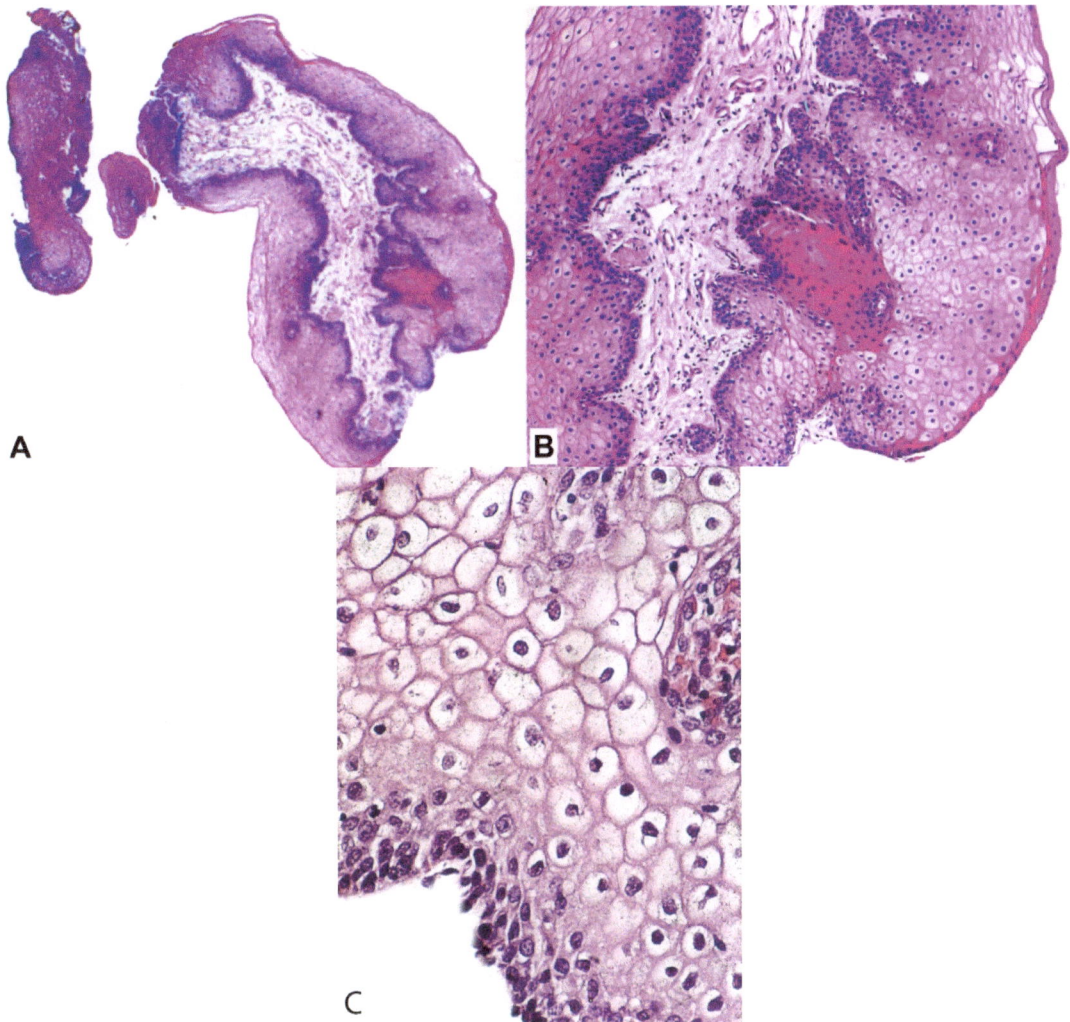

Figure 12 Papilloma of vocal cord (A, B) with significant koilocytosis in the surface epithelium (C) at higher power the vacuolated cells display mild nuclear atypia and proliferation of basal cell layer

Morphologic Variants of Squamous Cell Carcinoma of Upper Aerodigestive Tract

Table 5 Conventional and Variants of squamous cell carcinoma of Upper Aerodigestive Tract (n = 5487) Authors' series (1970-2005)	
Conventional Squamous Cell carcinoma	5278 (96.2%)
Verrucuous Carcinoma	89 (1.62%)
Lymphoepithelial Carcinoma	76 (1.38%)
Spindle cell Carcinoma	24 (0.44%)
Adenosquamous carcinoma	07
Basaloid Squamous Carcinoma	10
Papillary Squamous Carcinoma	02
Acantholytic Squamous Carcinoma	01

Conventional Squamous Cell Carcinoma:

This is the most common type of squamous carcinoma occurring in upper aero-digestive tract with 5285 cases out of 5487 total squamous carcinomas (96%, Table 5) diagnosed as conventional squamous cell carcinoma, as per our experience This is an easy histological diagnosis, which is rarely missed by a qualified pathologist with even limited experience (Figure 13 A, B). In some cases ,the primary is small and asymptomatic but cervical nodes display massive metastasis (Figure 13 C) Diagnosis of squamous cell carcinoma on a relatively small biopsy may be difficult, since mucosal reaction to granulomatous inflammation or some benign lesions may simulate squamous carcinoma (Figure 14). There are a variety of morphological variants of squamous cell carcinoma, which display a spectrum of biological behavior and are described below (14).

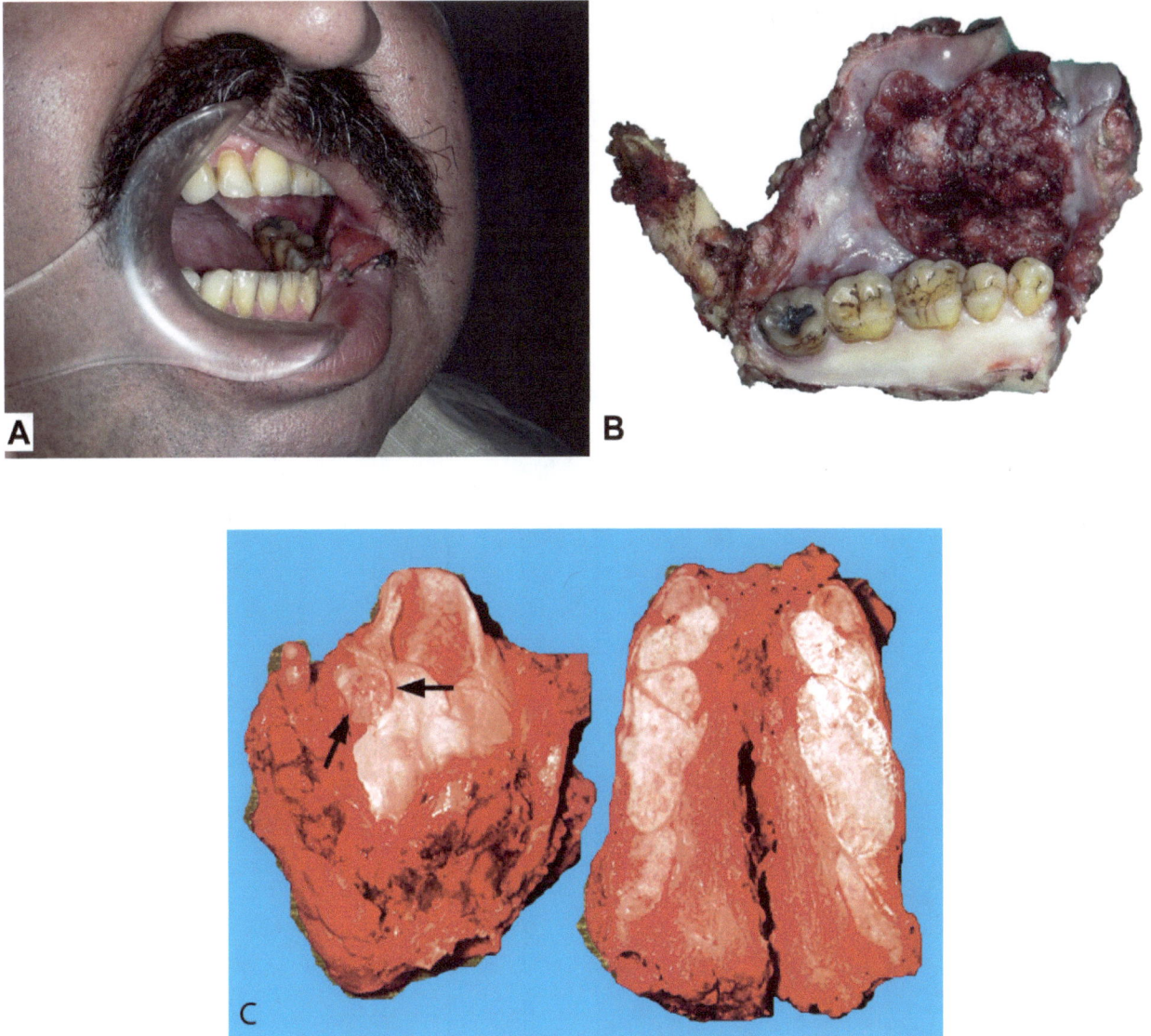

Figure 13 (A, B) Conventional squamous cell carcinoma of piriform fossa, ulcerated nodular growth (C) A < 1 cm flat extra-laryngeal growth (arrows), large metastases in cervical nodes

Pseudo epitheliomatous Change Versus Well differentiated Squamous cell carcinoma

It is not uncommon to come across oral mucosal lesions which may be over diagnosed as well differentiated squamous cell carcinoma. It is frequently observed in association with long standing ulcerative lesion with florid proliferation of keratinized squamous cells, often accompanied by plenty of chronic inflammatory reaction (Figure 14 A). A case of granular cell tumor of tongue is seen associated with pseudo epitheliomatous lesion completely mimicking a keratinized invasive squamous cell carcinoma (Figure 14 B, C, D).

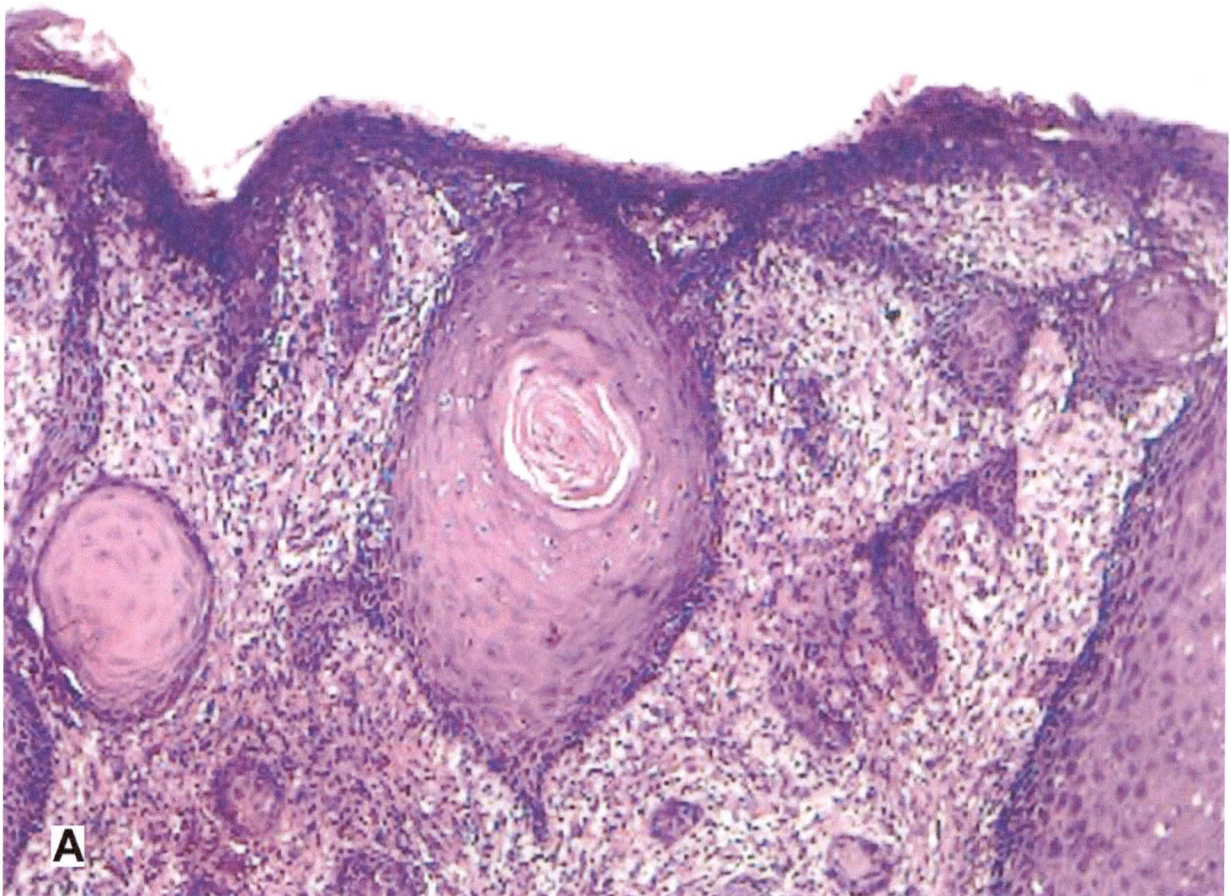

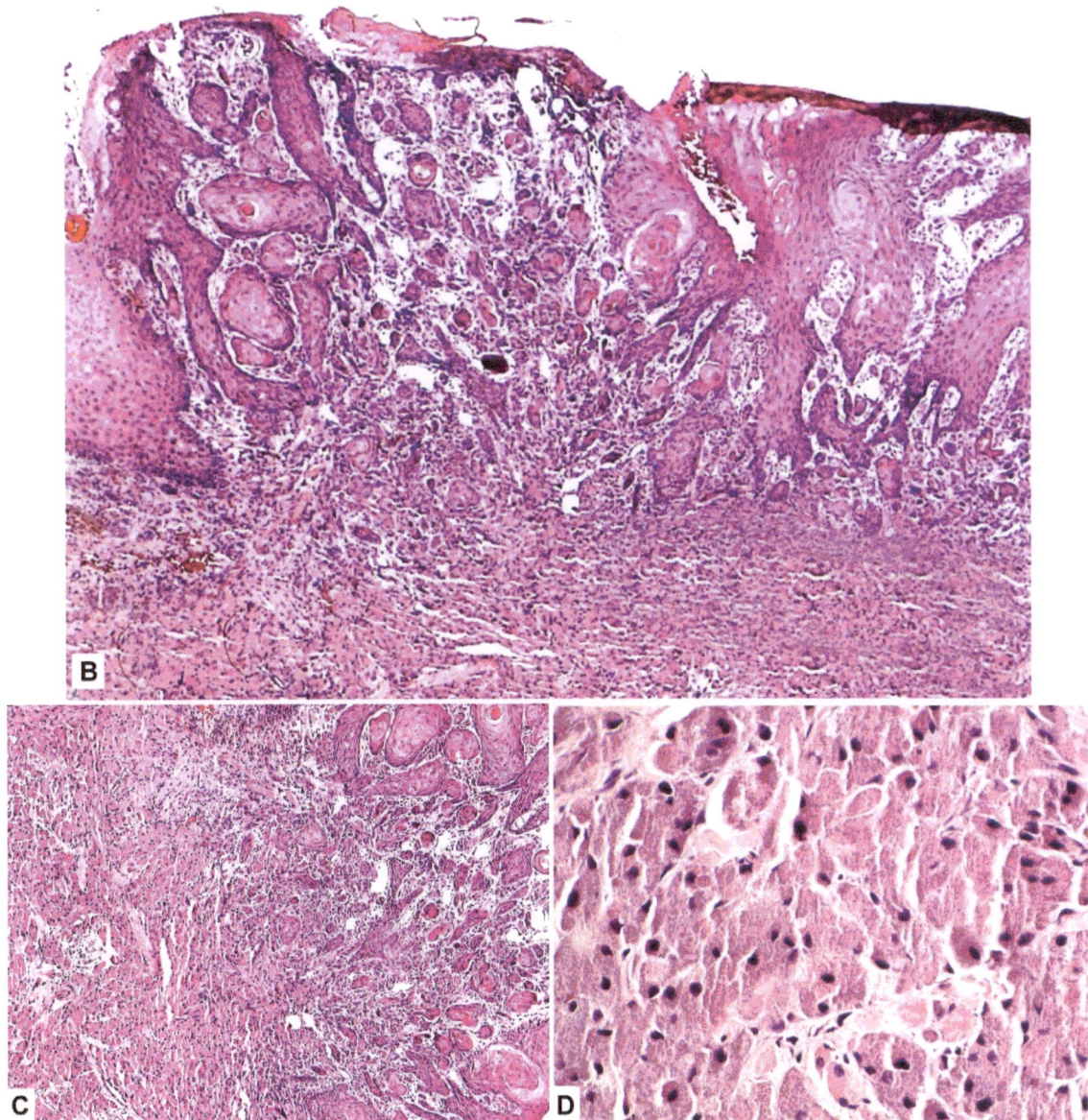

Figure 14 (A) pseudo epitheliomatous hyperplasia in a case of chronic gingivitis; (B&C) extensive pseudo carcinomatous proliferation in the mucosa of tongue overlying a granular cell tumor, granular tumor is at the left 1/3rd portion of (C); note sheets of large acidophilic granular cells; a biopsy from this lesion was interpreted s invasive squamous cell carcinoma on frozen section elsewhere and hemi-glossectomy performed

Micro invasive Carcinoma (Synonyms: superficial or "early" invasive carcinoma)

It is difficult to precisely define micro invasive carcinoma and its interpretation can be subjective. The lesion has been variously defined as: scattered isolated malignant cells in the upper sub epithelial zone or discrete foci of malignant cells invading through the basement membrane up to a depth of 2 mm or less from basement membrane (Figure 15). For micro invasive squamous carcinoma of cervix, the cut off point for depth of invasion is 3 mm. Whatever may be the definition, this diagnosis rules out lesion confined to mucosa (CIS/severe dysplasia) and those invading muscle or deeper structures. Histologically, microinvasive squamous carcinoma can develop as a continuation of severe dysplasia or CIS or can arise from a near normal squamous mucosa, directly dropping off from basal cell layer. The tumor nests tend to induce edema, fibrosis, inflammation or granulation tissue.

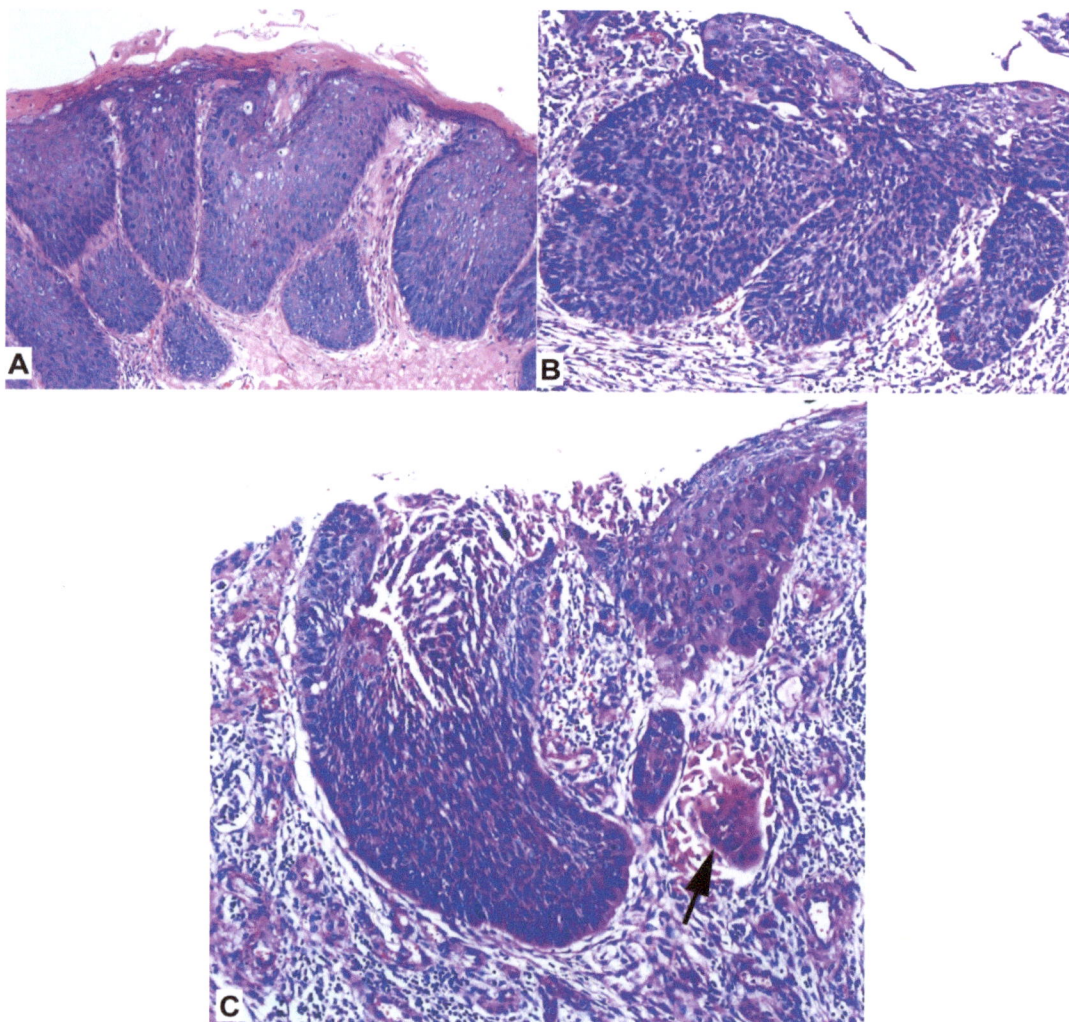

Figure 15 (A, B) Micro invasive squamous cell carcinoma: all illustrations show severe dysplasia to CIS in the surface epithelium with minimal invasion into fibrous inflammatory submucosa, the depth of penetration in this case was less than 1 mm; (C) Note neoplastic keratinized squamous island (arrow)

Reverse maturation with peripheral increased acidophilic cytoplasm as noted in Figure 15 (arrow) is often a good helpful criteria to make the diagnosis of microinvasive carcinoma. Microinvasive carcinoma is a biologically malignant tumor capable of metastasis if lymphovascular invasion is present. In fact, presence of lymphovascular invasion excludes a diagnosis of microinvasive carcinoma.

Human papilloma virus & carcinoma of Upper Aero-digestive tract (UADT)

HPV is the etiological agent responsible for most squamous carcinomas of the lower female genital tract and anus. It is also the cause of approximately 50 percent of penile squamous carcinomas. In immuno compromised patients HPV has been found to be associated with some cases of cutaneous squamous carcinomas.

In the last 20 years many published reports have shown a significant role for HPV in the development of head and neck cancers. It has been estimated that 20 to 25 percent of squamous carcinomas of upper aero-digestive tract are related to HPV infection. p16 immunostain as a surrogate marker has been used to assess HPV status in many institutions.. A widespread use of PCR and in situ hybridization in the detection of HPV has greatly facilitated more conclusive and confirmatory results.

HPV associated carcinoma occurs all throughout the aero-digestive tract, but majority arise within oropharynx, mainly base of tongue and palatine tonsils. These tumors have non-keratinizing or basaloid phenotype and occur in younger population. Patients having HPV associated squamous carcinoma have better outcome with improved overall survival and fewer recurrences as compared to tumors unrelated to HPV infection. Therefore, it is important to carry out immunohistochemical demonstration of p16 over-expression and HPV status (by PCR or in situ hybridization) to find out HPV relation to cases of SCC of UADT (15, 16)

Verrucous Carcinoma

This is a highly differentiated variant of squamous cell carcinoma, locally destructive but lacks metastatic capabilities. The prevalence of verrucous carcinoma (VC) is highest in oral cavity (17) and the incidence in our experience is 89 cases of VC among 5487 (1.62%) squamous cell carcinomas of UADT. Clinically the tumor is a large papillary non-ulcerated mass attached with a broad base to the mucosa. It is composed of nodular (cobble stone) papillary folds separated by deep clefts (Figure 16). The lesion tends to spread laterally than by deeper invasion (Figure. 17). However, as it extends into surface area it also can invade contiguous structures, including bone. The regional nodes are often enlarged and tender but this is usually due to infection and not metastases. Histologically, the tumor is a locally invasive warty growth with dense keratotic layer and sharply circumscribed pushing margins. This feature easily differentiates VC from the conventional low grade SCC. A band of chronic inflammation is almost always present at the base of the lesion.

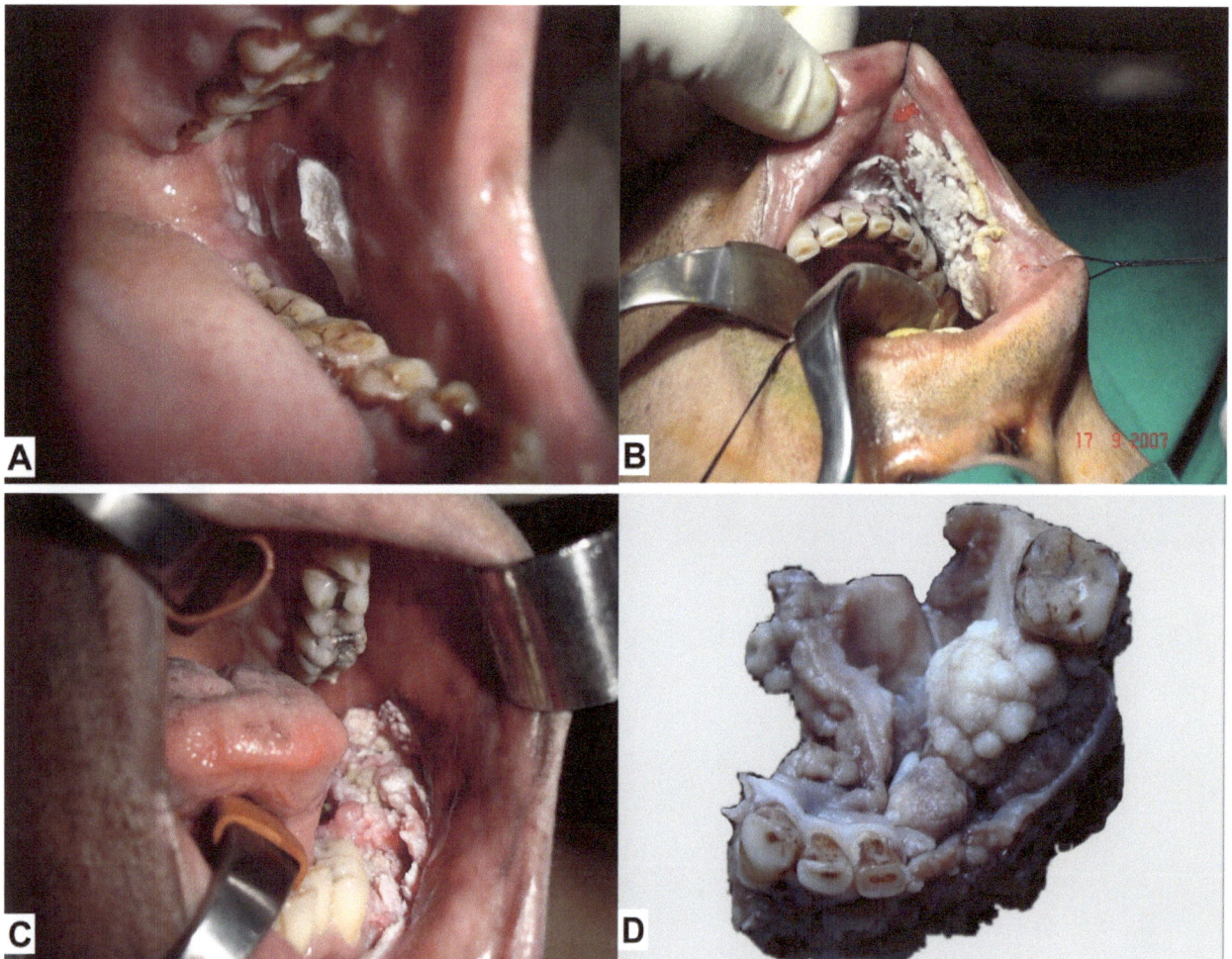

Figure 16 (A, B, C, D) Verrucous squamous carcinoma: the characteristic gross diagnostic features

Due to the extensiveness of the disease accompanied by palpable cervical nodes radical neck dissection has been carried out in some cases without tissue diagnosis of metastasis in cervical node. The nodes always show follicular hyperplasia and other reactive changes. Even non-caseating granulomas are encountered. The tumor may grow in the proximity of lymph nodes but almost never metastasizes to lymph nodes.

The most frequent sites of occurrence include oral cavity and larynx (Figures 17, 19). It occurs less commonly on the skin of foot and very rarely within a nasal sinus (Figure 20, 21). Histologically, VC has "benign appearing" squamous cell proliferation with following characteristics: uniform mature keratinocytes without dysplasia, lack of mitotic activity, massive surface keratinization and bulbous rete ridges with pushing margins (Figure 18a-b, 19). The pathological diagnosis is indeed difficult requiring multiple biopsies over a long period several years before the diagnosis is arrived at. The gross clinical appearance of VC is characteristic and the author has found it very informative to examine the patient in office. For the gross pictures shown in Figures 16 and 17 diagnosis of VC should be given even if the biopsy evidence is equivocal.

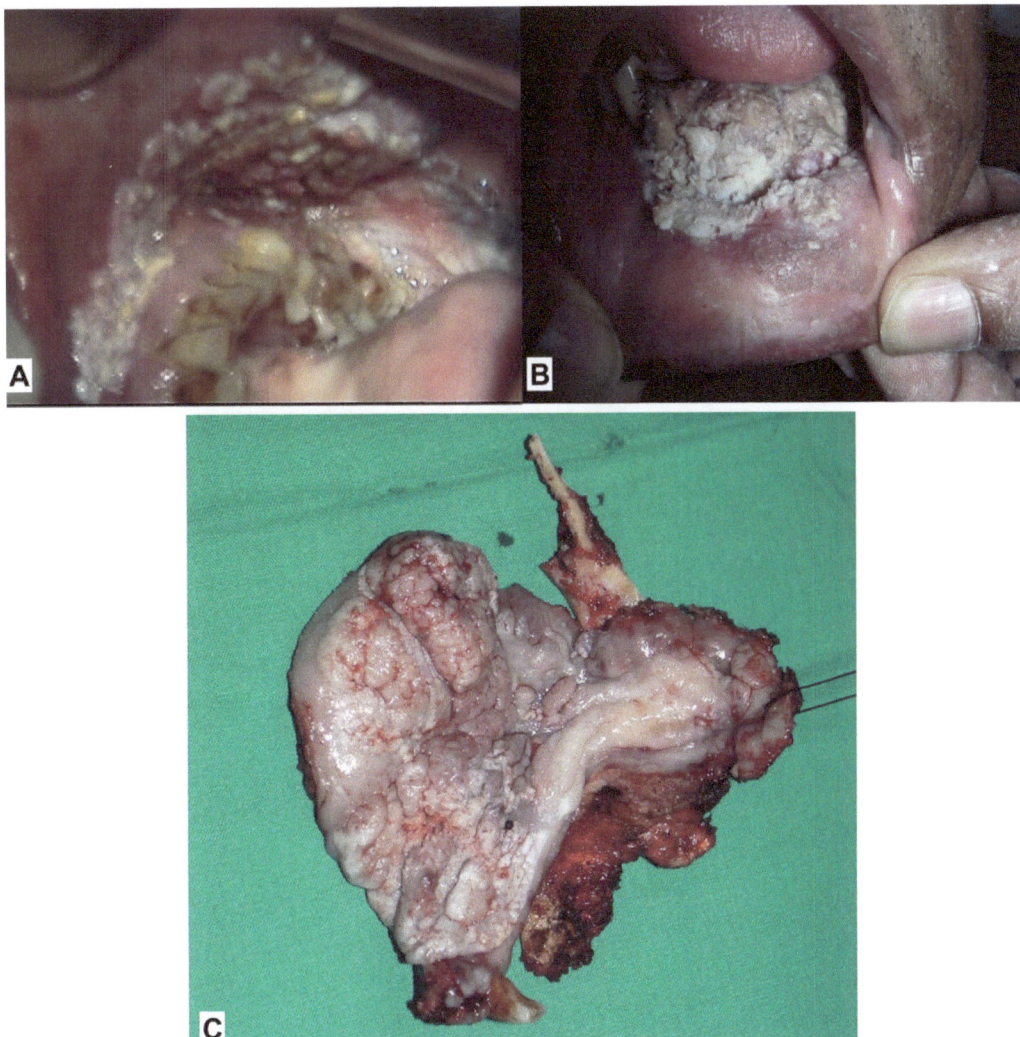

Figures 17 Verrucous carcinoma: (A) laterally spreading growth, (B) growth of flour of mouth spreading to lower lip, (C) extensive carcinoma of cheek, a flat nodular focally warty growth,

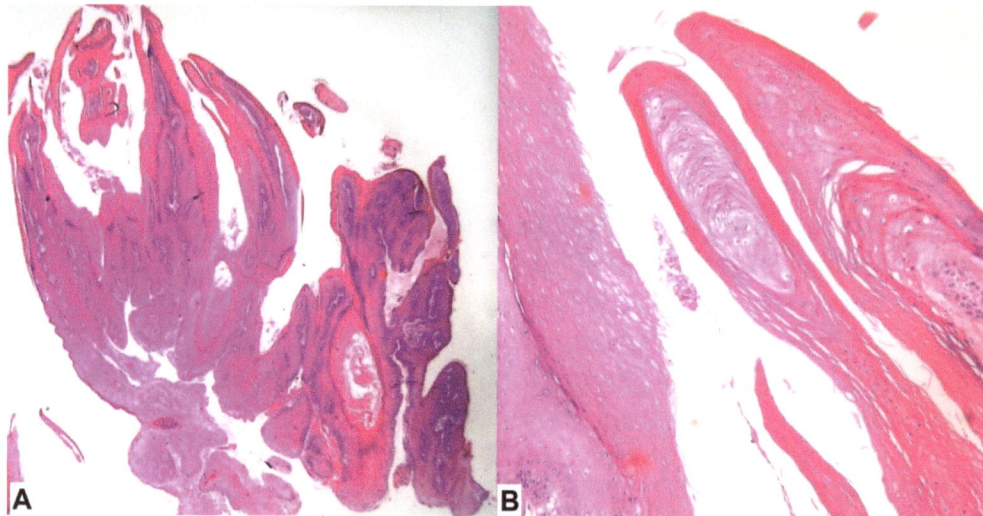

Figure 18a Verrucous carcinoma of cheek: exophytic, heavily keratinized growth, no nuclear anaplasia; one would hesitate to label this lesion as carcinoma without the knowledge of the gross appearance.

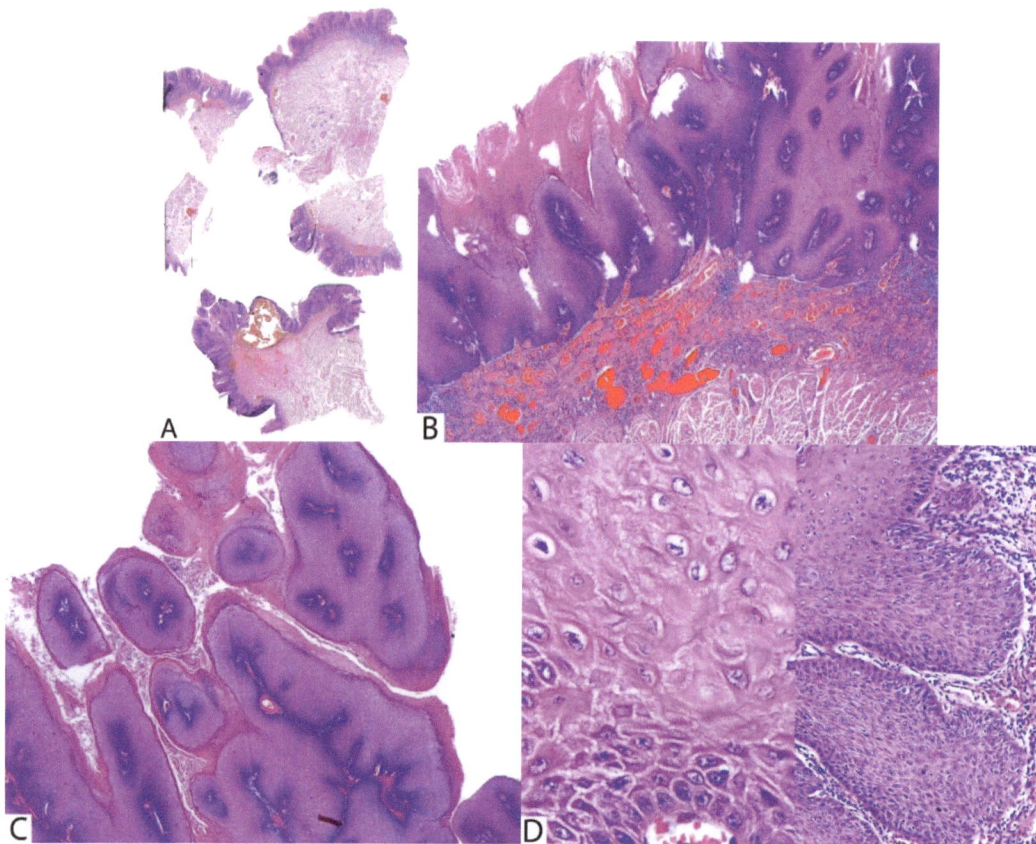

Fig 18b Verrucous carcinoma of cheek: (A) exophytic, keratinized growth, growing laterally along mucosal surface; (B) heavily keratinised exophytic growth (C) formation of papillary fronds (D) no nuclear anaplasia is seen in the superficial or the deeper part of the lesion; one would hesitate to label this lesion as carcinoma without the knowledge of the gross appearance.

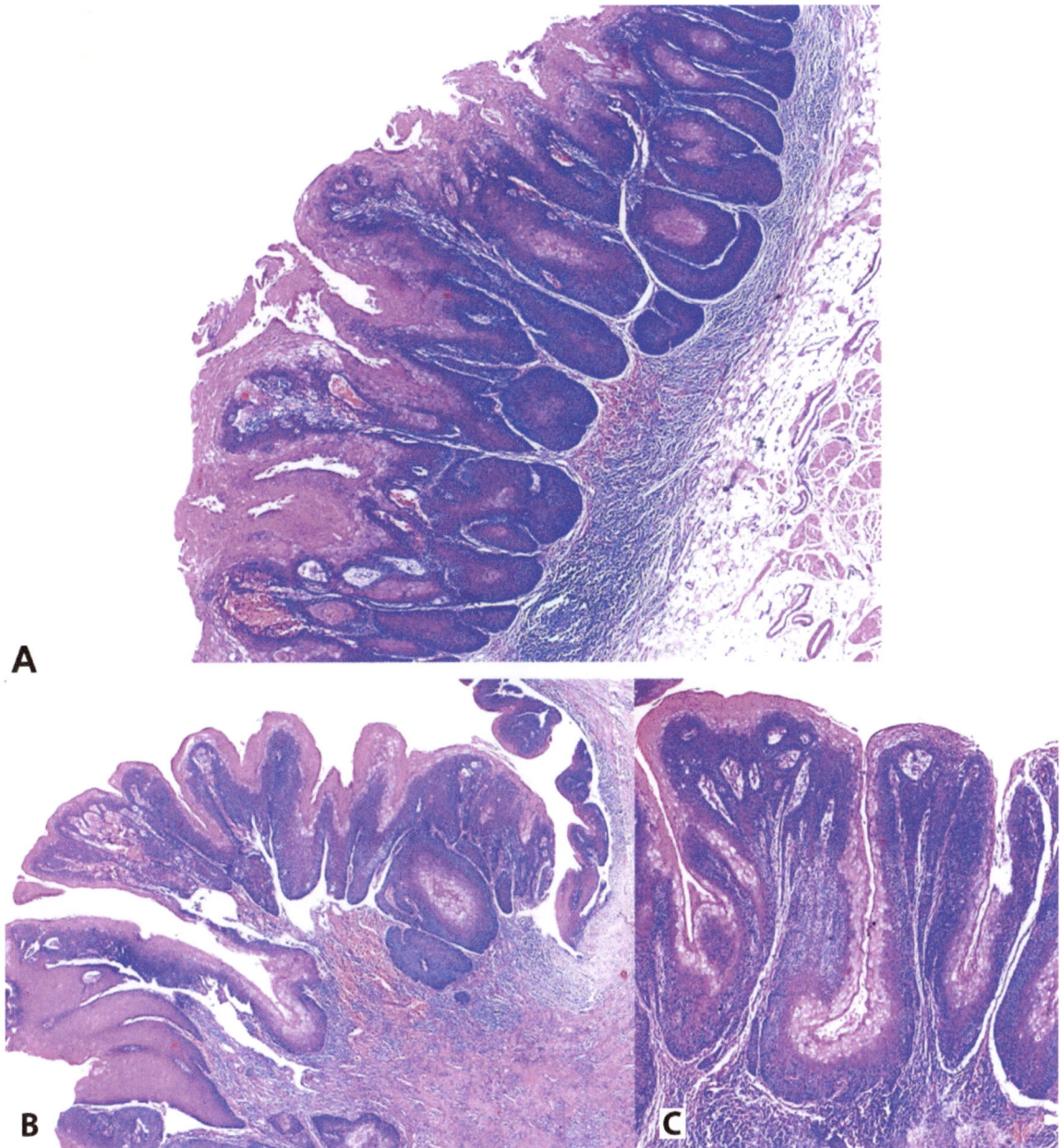

Figure 19 Verrucous carcinoma of supraglottic larynx: (A) hyperkeratotic minimally invasive growth with pushing margins note conspicuous basal cell proliferation with no nuclear anaplasia (B, C). The tumor has tendency to grow along the mucosal surface

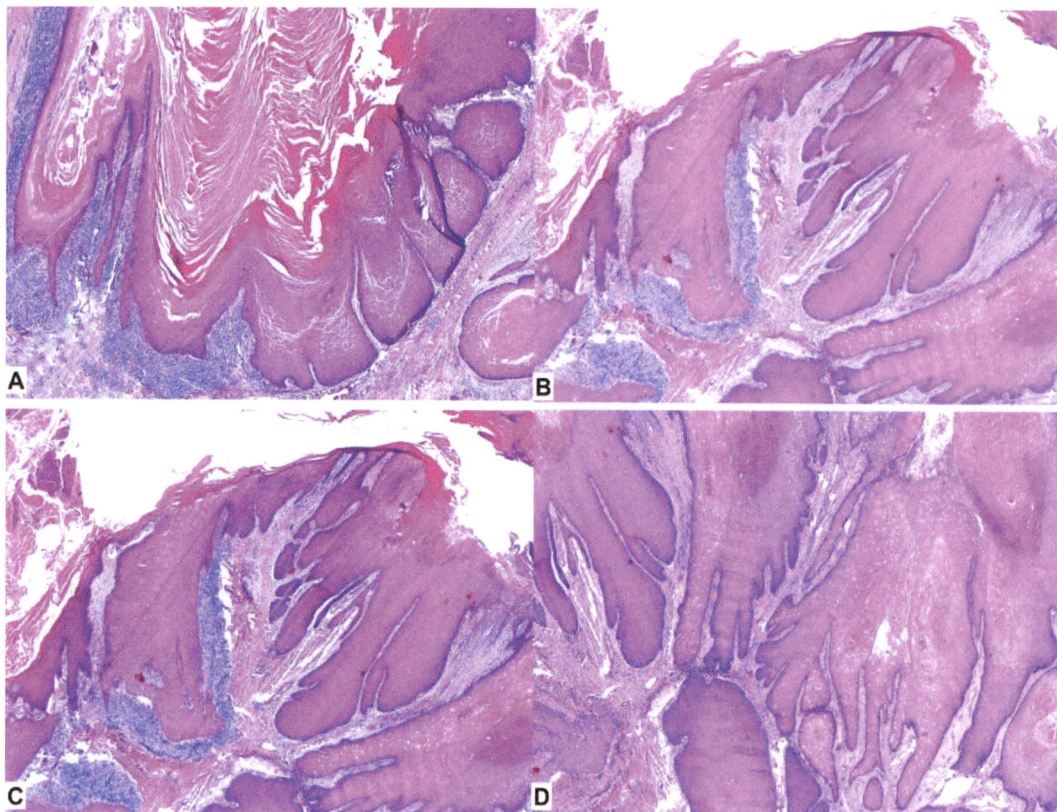

Figure 20 Carcinoma cuniculatum of foot: (A, B, C, D) massive proliferation of well differentiated squamous epithelium with excess keratinisation and broad deeply infiltrating processes without nuclear atypia, this tumor recurred with infiltration deep into the bones requiring amputation of forefoot

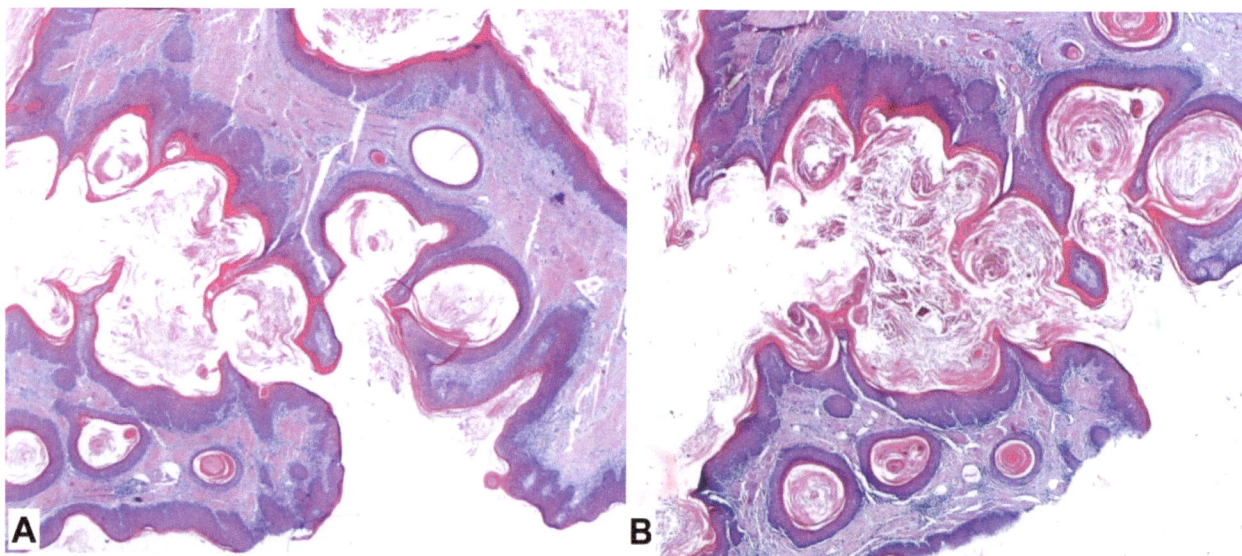

Figure 21 Verrucous carcinoma) involving and filling the maxillary sinus, an extremely rare occurrence (A, B), the bony sinus wall was intact

Nasopharyngeal carcinoma

(Synonyms: undifferentiated carcinoma of nasopharyngeal type, undifferentiated carcinoma with lymphoid stroma, Lymphoepithelioma, Lymphoepithelioma- like carcinoma and lymphoepithelial Carcinoma)

According to the WHO classification (2005) nasopharyngeal carcinoma (NPC) is defined as "A carcinoma arising in the nasopharyngeal mucosa that shows light microscopic or ultrastructural evidence of squamous differentiation." The current WHO classification (2005) is based on combination of anatomic and histologic features i.e. NPC with 4 distinct histologic subtypes.
Squamous cell carcinoma
Non-keratinizing squamous carcinoma
Differentiated non-keratinizing squamous carcinoma
Undifferentiated carcinoma
Basaloid squamous cell carcinoma

The subdivisions of NPC have clinical and therapeutic relevance with subtle morphologic correlations and molecular basis. It should be noted that the term lymphoepithelioma is a misnomer, for this cancer is entirely epithelial in origin with a secondary lymphoid component. The tumors usually involve the lateral wall of the nasopharynx, especially common in the fossa of Rosen Muller. The gross appearance of NPC varies from a mucosal bulge with intact surface epithelium to a clinically evident infiltrative growth to a totally unidentifiable lesion fortuitously sampled and histologically diagnosed as NPC.

The conventional keratinizing carcinoma will show intercellular bridges, dyskeratosis and keratinization. It is graded as moderately or poorly differentiated. About 25% of NPC cases are of this type.

The non-keratinizing NPC is a solid cellular growth with cohesive sheets of neoplastic cells, whose squamous origin is easily identified without the need for ancillary tests like immunohistochemistry or electron microscopy.

The undifferentiated type represents approximately 60% of all NPC cases and most frequently encountered in pediatric age groups. The tumor cells are characterized by mitotically active large round vesicular nuclei, prominent acidophilic nucleoli and scanty cytoplasm. A variable number of lymphocytes and fewer plasma cells are found intimately mixed with undifferentiated carcinoma cells. The lymphoplasmacytic infiltrate may be scanty or large enough to obscure the neoplastic cells. The other inflammatory cell types that may be present are eosinophils in large numbers and neutrophils. The carcinoma cells may have cohesive syncitial pattern (Regaud pattern) or a diffuse non-cohesive pattern (Schminke pattern). The diffuse pattern is the one, which is difficult to differentiate from malignant lymphoma on light microscopy (Figure 22 A, B). In this case, immunohistochemical staining can readily identify the epithelial origin of the neoplasm (Figure 23 & 24)). Trying to separate the non-keratinizing category into differentiated and undifferentiated is arbitrary and difficult to achieve. All subtypes of NPC are immunoreactive to cytokeratins including pan keratin and high molecular weight keratins. The overall 5-year survival for keratinizing type is about 25% and approximately 65% for both the non-keratinizing types. This apparent paradox can be explained by the fact that the undifferentiated non-keratinizing types are far more radiosensitive than keratinizing type of nasopharyngeal carcinoma (18).

Undifferentiated carcinoma of nasopharynx is known to be associated with the EB virus and its endemic geographical distribution, particularly among residents of south East Asia and Eskimos. EBV has an etiological role in the genesis of NPC as shown by in situ hybridization studies. In the last 20 years, this tumor has been reported with increasing frequency in sites other than nasopharynx, including upper aero-digestive tract, sinonasal tract, salivary glands, lung, thymus, stomach, skin, breast, uterine cervix, vagina and urinary bladder. And quite naturally this has led to a belief that EBV may be associated with tumors with lymphoepithelial morphology, regardless of the location (19).

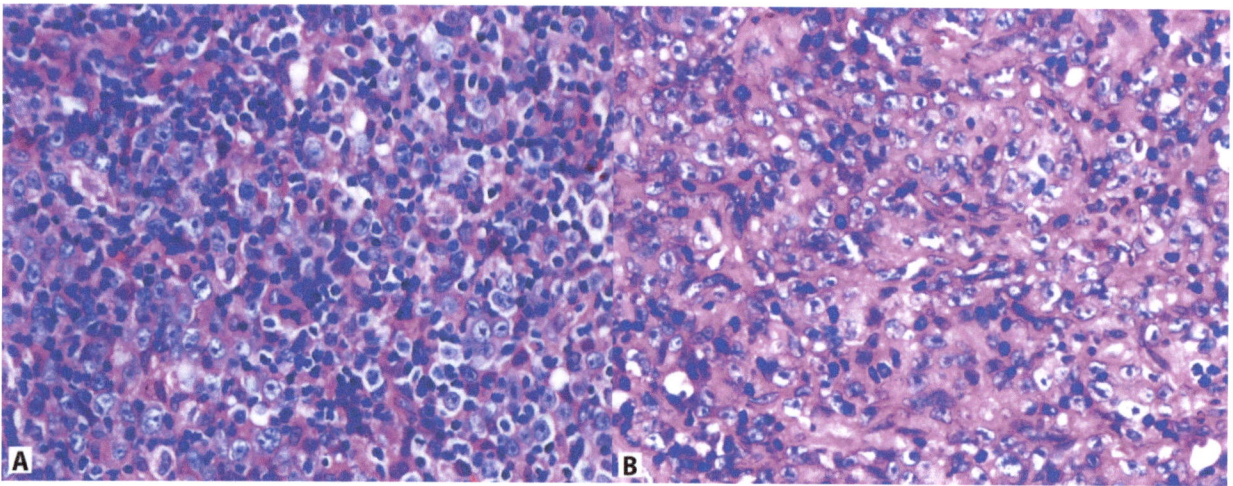

Figure 22 undifferentiated carcinoma of nasopharynx (A&B): epithelial cells have large nuclei and prominent nucleoli & lymphocytes show dark nuclei. NHL cannot be ruled out without IHC.

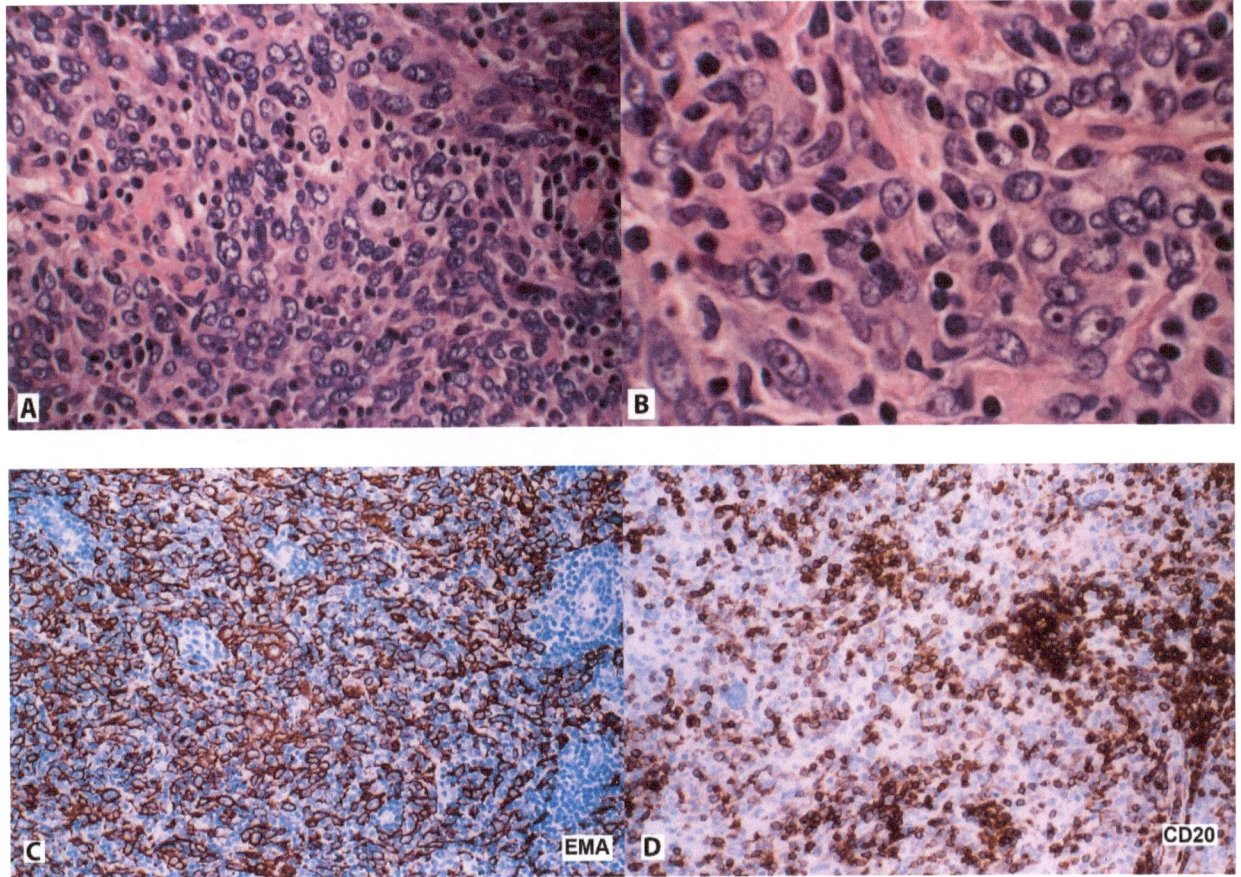

Figure 23 Undifferentiated nasopharyngeal carcinoma, lymphepithlioma-like (A & B): intimate mixture of epithelial and lymphocytic cells. (C) EMA decorates epithelial cells), (D) CD20 stains the lymphocytes

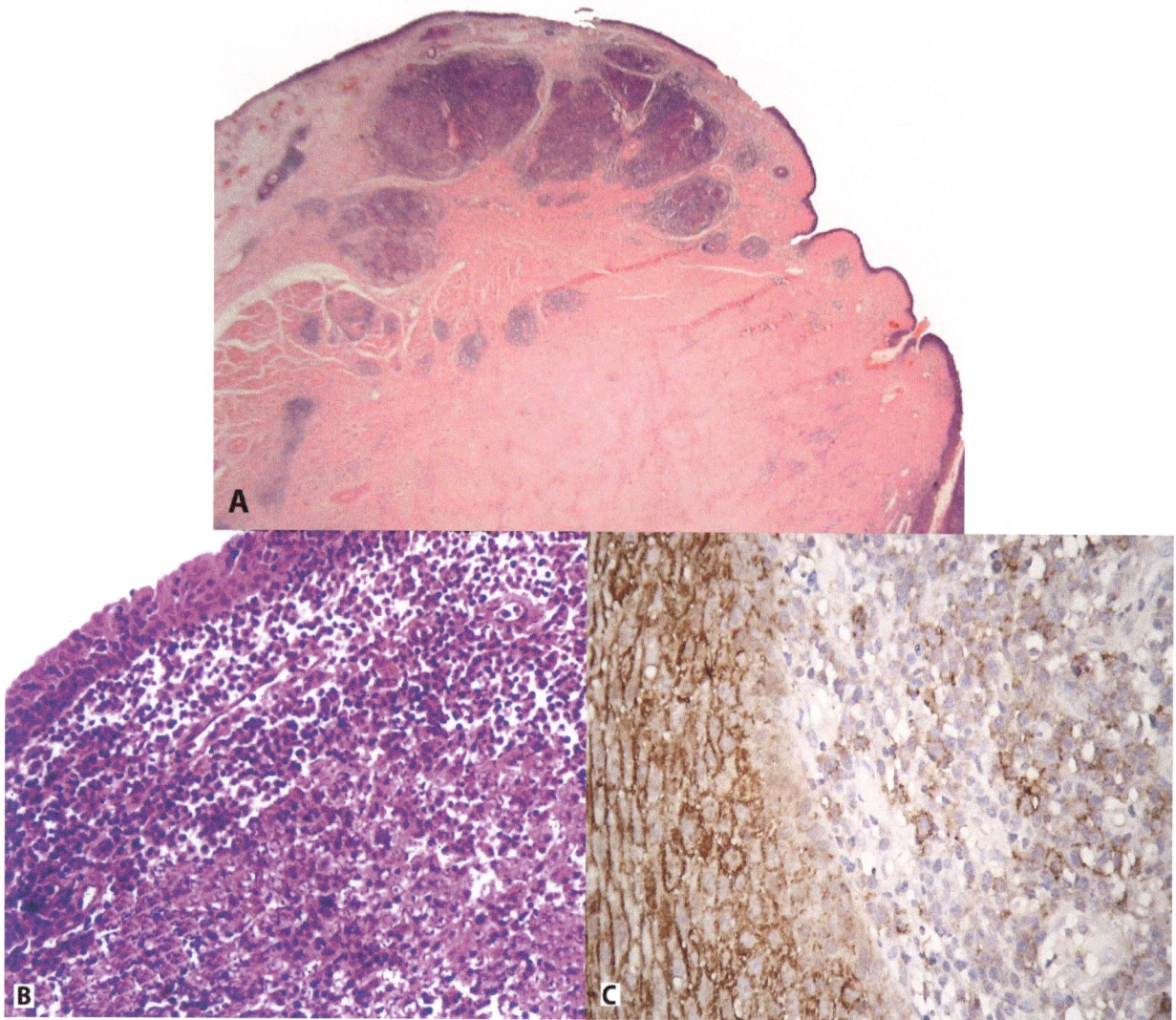

Figure 24 (A) Low power view of tumor in vocal cord (B) undifferentiated tumor with overlying normal squamous mucosa (C) EMA decorates the epithelial cells but not the lymphocytes the stained squamous mucosal on the left serves as a normal control

Spindle Cell (sarcomatoid) Squamous cell carcinoma

(Synonyms: carcinosarcoma, squamous cell carcinoma with sarcomatous stroma, metaplastic carcinoma, collision tumor, pseudosarcoma, polypoid squamous cell carcinoma etc)

These are rare tumors and accounted for only 24 cases out of 5487 (0.44%) squamous carcinomas of aero-digestive tract in our experience. Grossly, the lesion is a polypoid exophytic or fungating mass that occurs at various sites in head and neck in order of decreasing frequency: larynx, oral cavity, hypopharynx (piriform fossa), sinonasal tract and oropharynx.

Not infrequently, spindle cell carcinoma poses a challenge in classification, diagnosis and

treatment. The tumor comprises poorly differentiated spindle cell proliferation and component of conventional squamous cell carcinoma (Figure 25).The latter may include invasive differentiated squamous carcinoma or even an in situ squamous carcinoma in the mucosa. In many cases, ulceration of the surface of the tumor may destroy the diagnostic squamous carcinoma component. The sarcomatoid component is predominantly spindle cell type with fascicular, palisading or storiform growth patterns. Pleomorphic cells with bizarre nuclear forms, prominent nucleoli and abnormal mitoses are almost always present. Giant cells, whether multinucleated, foreign body type or osteoclast type are present in some cases, dispersed throughout the neoplasm.

Nearly 60% of spindly cells are cytokeratin immunoreactive and ultrastructurally, display evidence of epithelial differentiation in the form of desmosomes and tonofilaments. In some cases (<10%), sarcomatous transformation can be so complete that malignant cartilage; bone or muscle cells are formed. Several mesenchymal markers are focally expressed: smooth muscle actin- 33%; S-100 protein - 5% and desmin- <2% occur. Other markers like HMB-45, chromogranin, GFAP are not expressed. As alluded to earlier, the carcinomatous part of the tumor may be destroyed or so miniscule that it may be totally missed. This can pose a diagnostic problem and a battery of 8 cytokeratin makers will have to be tested. A short cost effective panel of AE1/AE3, epithelial membrane antigen, CK1 and CK18 has been recommended for a definitive diagnosis of spindle cell (sarcomatous) squamous carcinoma (20, 21)

The underlying events associated with the development of spindle cell carcinoma and the biological significance is not known. It is now accepted that sarcomatous component is part of the tumor and fully capable of metastasis and is not just a reactive change.

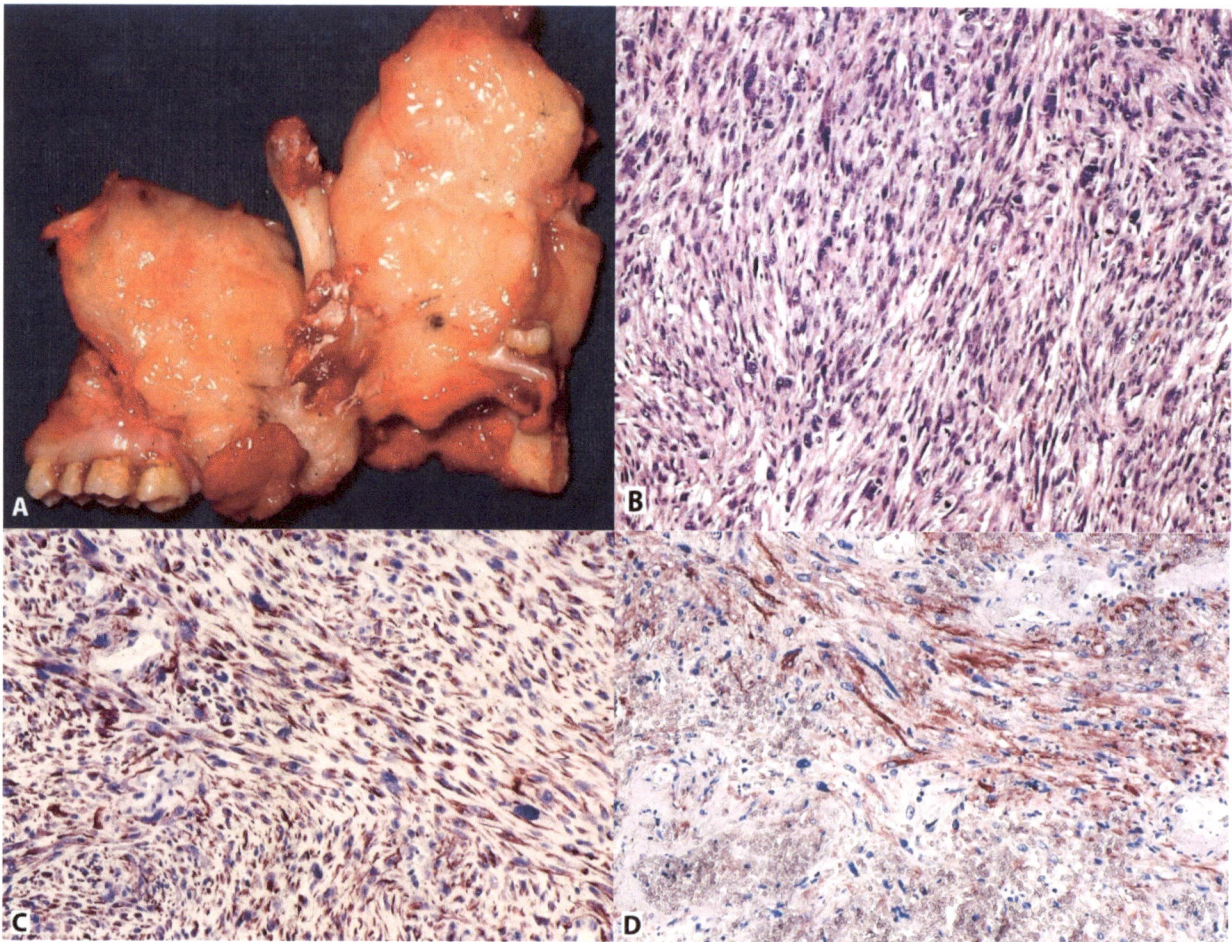

Figure 25: (A)Polypoid mass in mouth, (B) a pleomorphic high grade spindle sarcoma (C) Cytokeratin positive spindly cells (D) immunostaing of HHF-35 in spindle cells(smooth muscle cells)

Adenosquamous carcinoma

A rare aggressive variant of SCC arises from the surface epithelium and is characterized by conventional SCC and true Adenocarcinoma (22). The tumor is encountered in any part of oral cavity and oropharynx but has been most commonly reported from tongue, flour of mouth and tonsillar pillars. The two components occur in close proximity, but tend to be discrete and separate (Figure 26), not intermingled like mucoepidermoid carcinoma. The SCC component presents as an in situ or invasive carcinoma. The adenocarcinoma component occurs in the deeper part of the tumor and is not of any specific type. It is characterized by tubular acini with intra luminal or intracellular mucin and even signet ring cells. Metastases display both elements, often in unequal proportion. The differential diagnosis includes mucoepidermoid carcinoma, acantholytic SCC, SCC invading minor salivary glands and necrotizing sialometaplasia. Little or no keratinization and diffuse intermingling pattern of mucin secreting and squamous cells is typical of mucoepidermoid carcinoma. The adenocarcinoma component in Adenosquamous carcinoma expresses CEA and CK 7. Adenosquamous carcinoma arises from basal cells of the surface epithelium, which is capable of a divergent differentiation.

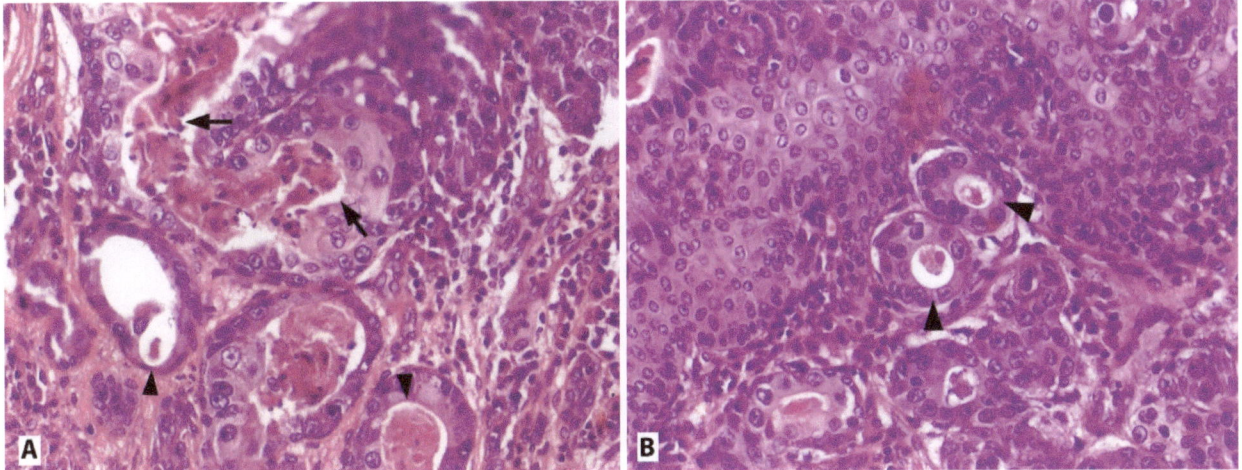

Figure 26 Adenosquamous carcinoma: (A) keratinized squamous carcinoma (arrows) (B) glandular component (arrow heads)

Basaloid Squamous Cell Carcinoma

(23, 24, 25, 25a)

The diagnosis of this basaloid squamous cell carcinoma vs non-keratinizing squamous cell carcinoma can be at times difficult, when keratinizing component is not identifiable. Basaloid squamous cell carcinoma, as defined by Wain's criteria, is intimately associated with keratinizing squamous cell carcinoma. Tumors are composed of a lobular proliferation of small, crowded cells with scant cytoplasm and round, hyperchromatic nuclei. Cystic spaces with mucin-like material, coagulative necrosis and stromal hyalinosis with basement membrane-like material are other findings (25a). This is an aggressive biphasic variant of SCC consisting of a high grade basaloid epithelial proliferation and traditional SCC, typically occurring at the base of tongue, piriform fossa, supraglottic larynx and tonsils. Other sites in oral cavity are involved less commonly. It presents at an advanced stage (III or IV) and follows an aggressive course. The major histological feature is the presence of solid cellular basaloid cell pattern intimately associated with squamous cell carcinoma, carcinoma in situ or focal squamous differentiation (23, 24). It consists of small crowded cells containing hyperchromatic pleomorphic nuclei, scanty cytoplasm, small cystic spaces, focal tumor necrosis and variable hyalinosis. In the first publication on the subject, 8 out of 10 cases had metastases in the nodes or other organs. . Basaloid squamous carcinoma is often associated with HPV infection, which is readily identified on IHC (Figure 27 A to E). The tumor should be differentiated from adenoid cystic carcinoma (25, 25a, 25b) and this is done on the basis of the following:

Basaloid SCC is in continuity with mucosa showing dysplasia / CIS with focal squamous islands, prominent nuclear anaplasia and diffuse p63 positivity.

Adenoid cystic carcinoma, shows none of these features except mild focal p63 expression.

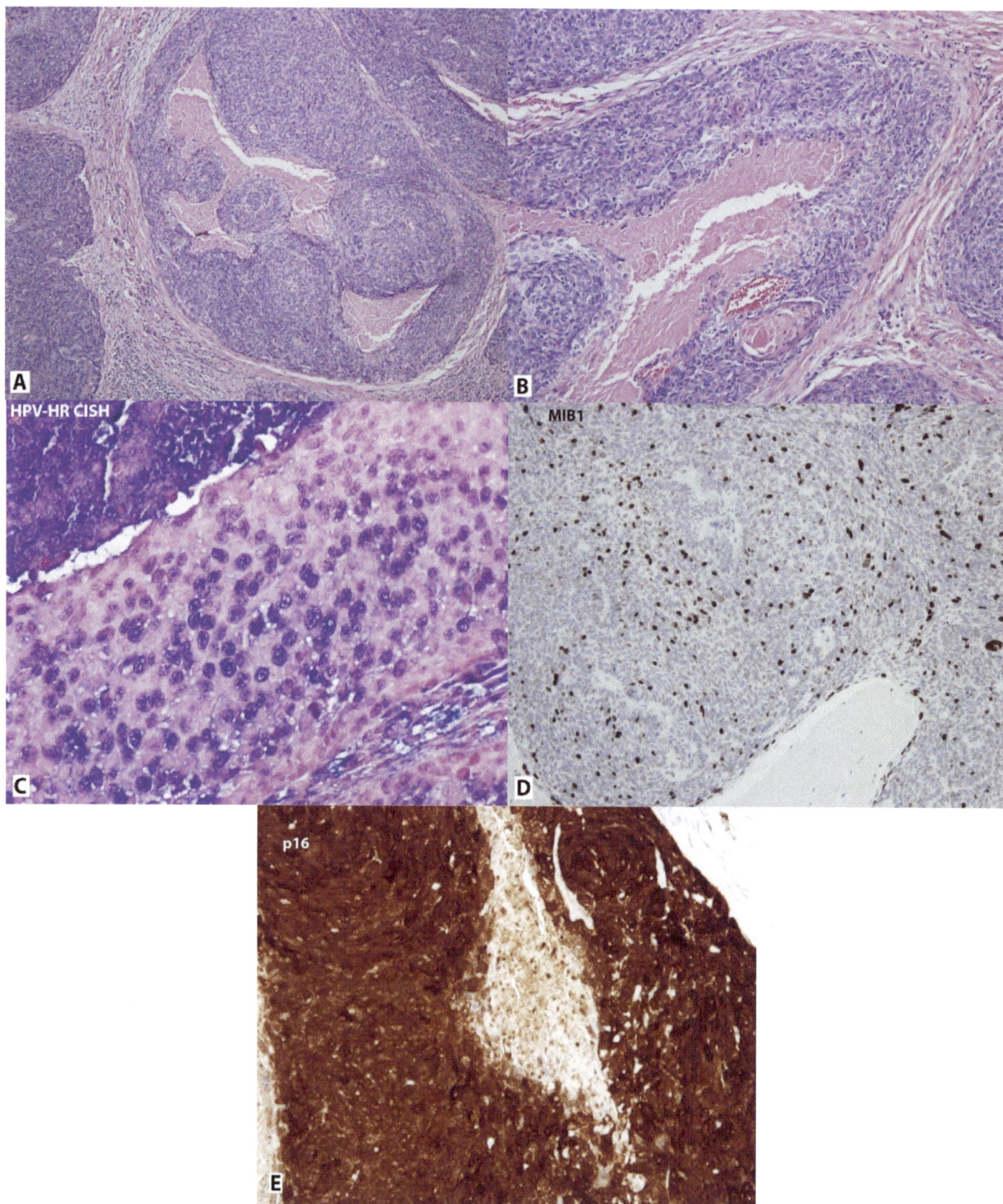

Figure 27 (A& B) basaloid squamous differentiation (C) demonstration of HPV virus by in situ hybridization (D) MIB1 shows high index of proliferation marker (E) p16 is diffusely and strongly expressed (marker for HPV)

Papillary Squamous cell carcinoma (PSCC)

This is an uncommon but distinct subtype of squamous cell carcinoma of UADT. It is most commonly located in larynx, oropharynx and sinonasal tract. The papillary pattern consists of multiple thin delicate, filliform, finger like papillary projections. The papillae are lined predominantly by non-keratinizing squamous cell carcinoma in situ that is similar to in situ squamous carcinoma of cervix, with full thickness lack of maturation and significant nuclear anaplasia (Figure 28). It is very difficult to determine presence of stromal invasion, particularly since the carcinomatous epithelium is usually of in situ type. However, a significant cell proliferation forming a clinically evident growth is beyond the concept of carcinoma in situ. There is consensus among surgical pathologists that papillary squamous carcinoma should be considered as invasive, even in the absence of definitive stromal invasion (26, 27). Differentiation of PSCC from verrucous carcinoma (VC) is not difficult. VC is distinguished from PSCC by its lack of nuclear atypia, high degree of cellular differentiation, marked surface keratinization and presence of pushing well defined margins. Nearly 70% of PSCC cases reveal p16 imunoreactivity and HPV by in situ hybridization, which strongly suggests an etiological role for HPV infection. As with other HPV associated cases of SCC, the majority of HPV associated (70%) PSCC have been oropharyngeal (base of tongue and tonsils) (28).

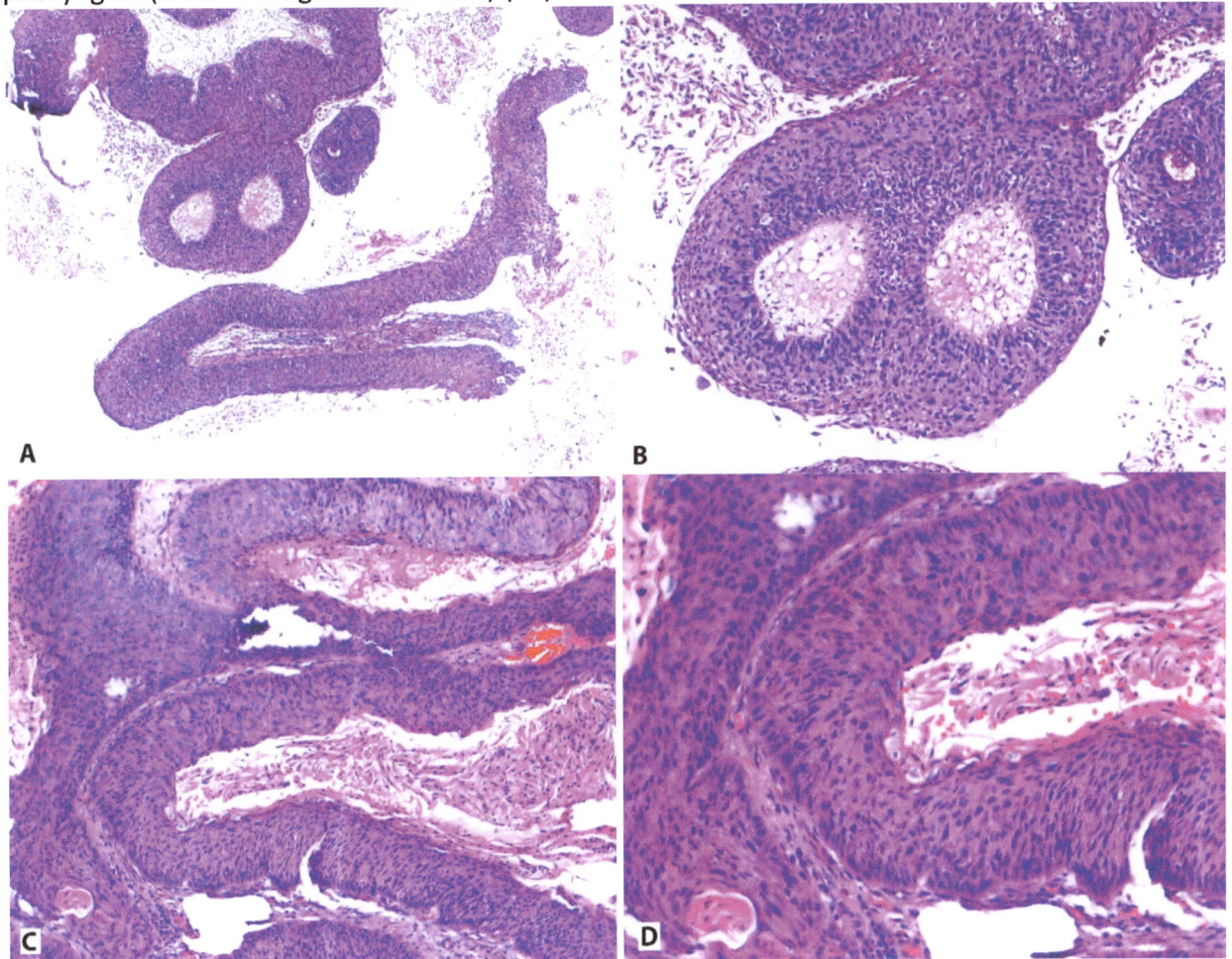

Figure 28 (A & B) scanner view of papillary squamous carcinoma, (C & D) higher magnification of the same tumor identifying squamous cell morphology)

Acantholytic squamous cell carcinoma (ASCC)

(Synonyms: adenoid squamous cell carcinoma, pseudoglandular SCC, pseudovascular adenoid squamous cell carcinoma, angiosarcoma like SCC etc)

This is an uncommon variant of SCC, which shows acantholysis of tumor cells creating pseudolumina and pseudoglandular differentiation. Study of large number of sections is required to detect an easily identifiable keratinized squamous component (Figure 29 A, B). Intra-tumor complex slit like spaces with a pseudo glandular or micro-acinar pattern is always present (Figure 29 C, D). The lining cells are medium sized polygonal or epithelioid in shape. It is important to know that angiosarcoma (particularly epithelioid type) of oral cavity has a strong histological resemblance to ASCC and immunohistochemical staining is necessary for differentiation. Standard epithelial and endothelial markers are usually adequate for accurate diagnosis. However, many workers have experienced difficulties in the immunohistochemical differentiation because in angiosarcoma cytokeratins are often well expressed and the plentiful vessels in the stroma of ASCC stained with endothelial markers may overwhelm ASCC cells expressing cytokeratins.

Recently, it has been shown that FLi-1 antibody immunostaining (typically nuclear) of the endothelial cells of angiosarcoma readily differentiated from the strong cytoplasmic stained epithelial cells with laminin-5 stain (29).

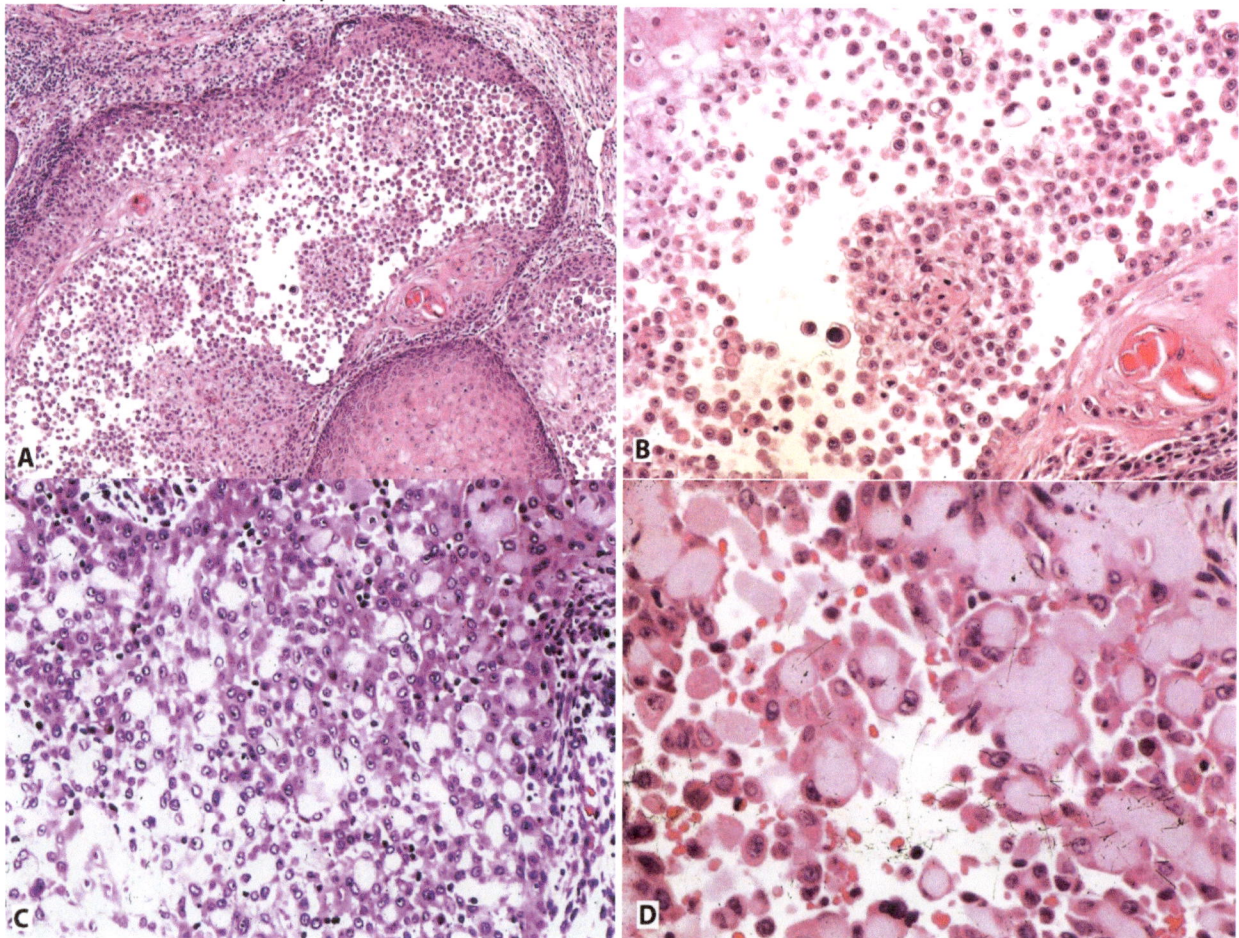

Figure 29 (A & B) a growth of squamous carcinoma with conspicuous acantholysis and rare focus of keratinization, (C & D) microacinar or pseudo glandular pattern

Lymphoproliferative lesions of Head & Neck

Lymphoproliferative lesions occur in nasopharynx, sinonasal tract and salivary glands and each of these sites is affected by different subsets of benign and neoplastic lymphoid proliferations. The type of lymphoma seen reflects the underlying biology of the particular site involved. The lymphoid tissue in the nasopharynx and Waldeyer's ring are functionally similar to the mucosa associated lymphoid tissue of gastrointestinal tract (malt). Most commonly low-grade B cell lymphomas occur at these sites, particularly mantle cell lymphoma. Lymphoid tissue does not naturally occur in the sinonasal tract but this is the site for natural killer (NK) T cell lymphoma, which is almost always associated with EB virus. Nasopharynx is the reservoir for EB virus but curiously lymphomas at this site do not contain EBV. Salivary glands do not harbor lymphoid tissue normally but it is the site predisposed to the acquisition of maltoma following appropriate antigenic stimulation.

Any type of lymphoma can occur in Head & Neck region but following lymphoproliferative lesions have particular site wise predilection and will be described here.

Table 6: Lymphoproliferative lesions of the head and neck	
Sinonasal tract:	Wegener's granulomatosis
	NK/T cell lymphoma
Salivary glands:	Lymphoepithelial sialadenitis (Sjogren's)
	Marginal zone B cell lymphoma
Nasopharynx:	Low grade B cell lymphomas (mantle cell)
Oral Cavity:	Lymphomatoid granulomatosis

Wegener's Granulomatosis

Wegener's granulomatosis (WG) is one of the anti-neutrophil cytoplasmic antibodies (ANCA) associated small vessel vasculitides and is distinguished by its predilection to affect the upper and lower respiratory tracts and kidneys clinically. It is histologically characterized by a triad of necrosis, granulomatous inflammation and vasculitis. However, in a large study of WG in head and neck region only 16% of cases had the diagnostic histological triad (30). And vasculitis, necrosis and granulomatous inflammation were found overall in 26%, 33%, and 42% respectively of all cases of head and neck WG. Other features of some diagnostic significance include micro abscesses and multinucleated giant cells scattered in a diffuse inflammatory infiltrate of neutrophils, plasma cells, lymphocytes and histiocytes. All these changes are encountered in many cases of infective granulomatous lesions and necrotizing inflammatory disorders with vasculitis. Thus, histological diagnosis of WG on the basis of inherently small sized nasal biopsies is indeed difficult or even impossible (30). A close correlation with clinical and laboratory findings is indispensable.

C-ANCA is positive in most patients of active classical WG with a sensitivity of 90% to 98%. Whereas sensitivity in limited or inactive disease varies from 65% to 70%, it is even much lower in cases of WG in remission. Although C-ANCA is positive in vast majority of cases of WG, it should not be used as a sole criterion in place of biopsy to arrive at a diagnosis. In about 25% of cases of WG perinuclear P-ANCA with MPO specificity is found. However, this test is more frequently positive in Churg-Strauss syndrome, microscopic polyarteritis, polyarteritis nodosa and vasculitis associated crescentic glomerulonephritis (31).

All typical clinical findings, particularly involvement of kidney are not present in all cases of nasal or pulmonary WG, since limited form of the disease exists, where only one organ like skin, lung, eye or oral mucosa may be involved. To differentiate WG from other conditions, a detailed study of the histological components of the triad is required. The vasculitic lesions involve capillaries, venules, arterioles, small arteries and veins. There is necrosis of the vessel wall and the angiocentric infiltrate ranges from being frankly granulomatous to neutrophil-predominant. Not uncommonly it is difficult to isolate intact vessels showing a well-defined vasculitic lesion. The nature of granulomatous lesion in WG should be clearly understood. A tight sarcoid type of granuloma is almost never found. Langhan's giant cell or foreign type giant cells are scattered at the periphery of the necrotic zone. In some cases, palisading histiocytes are found to outline the necrotic area. Necrosis is usually an irregularly shaped area and may show caseous type material, eosinophilic fibrinoid type of appearance or necrotic debris with abundant neutrophils (Figure 30 A to F) . It is obvious why differentiation from tuberculosis or other infective lesions can be so difficult in cases of Wegener's granulomatosis..

The NIH study (32) has proposed following criteria for diagnosis of WG in head and neck biopsies to be considered only after infective and other causes of midline granulomatous disease are ruled out (table 7-Head and neck= HN, Lung=L, Kidney=K).

Table 7: Criteria for diagnosis of WG in head and neck biopsies	
Definitive diagnosis	Vasculitis + granulomatous inflammation + necrosis & clinical involvement of HN, L & K
Definitive diagnosis	two major histological criteria & clinical involvement of HN, L,& K
Probable diagnosis	two major histological criteria & clinical involvement of only one of HN, L & K
Suggestive of WG	only one major histological criteria & clinical involvement of HN, L & K
No diagnosis of WG	None of major histological criteria even if clinical involvement of HN, L & K

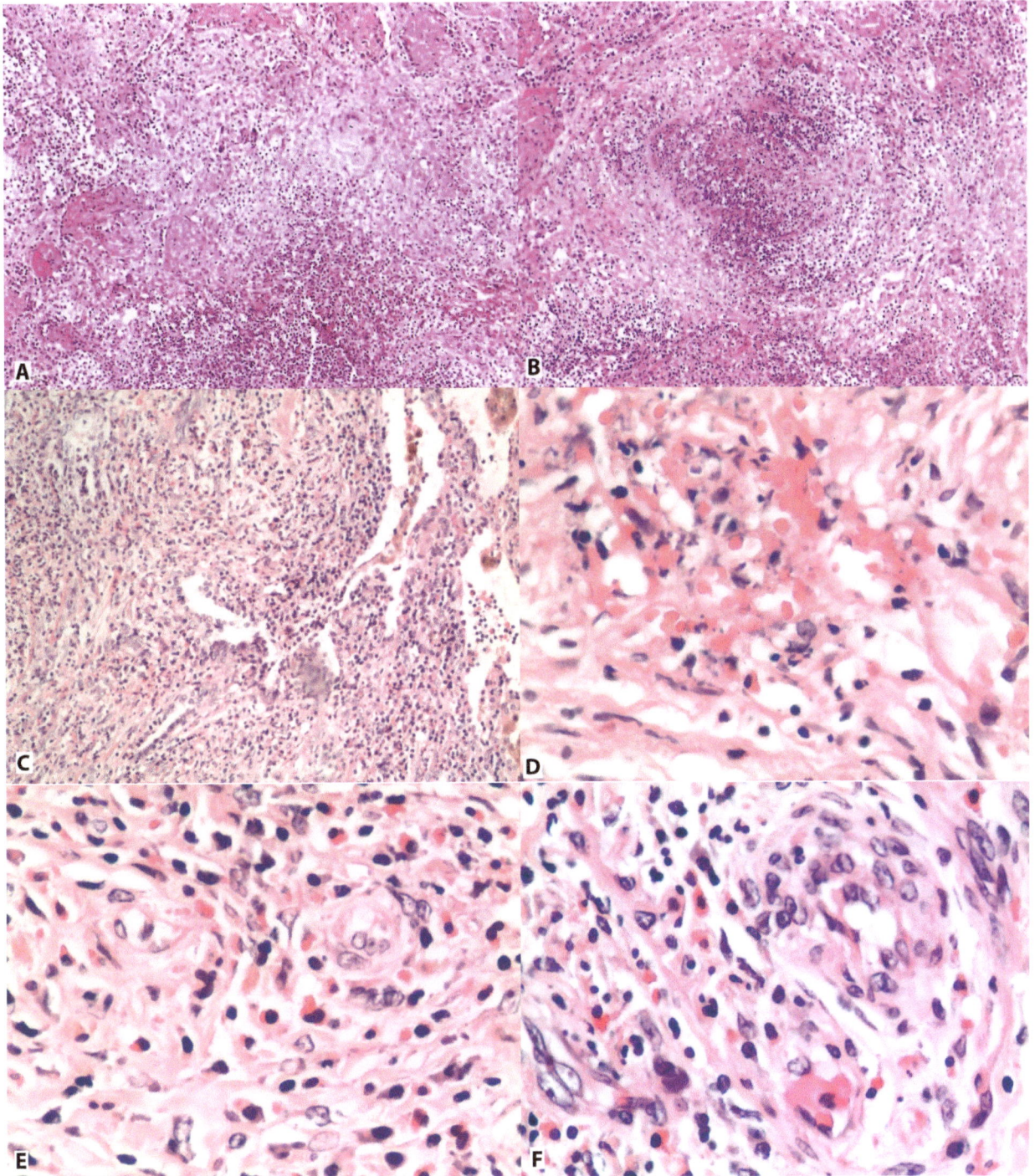

Figure 30 (A & B) ill defined granulomatous inflammation (C) diffuse subacute inflammation (D) focal necrosis with neutrophils (E & F) small vessel vasculitis with eosinophilia

NK/T cell Lymphoma Of Sinonasal Tract

The sinonasal tract does not contain lymphoid tissue and yet extra nodal NK/T cell lymphoma is most frequently encountered in this anatomical region. In this section only NK/T cell lymphoma and lymphomatoid granulomatosis will be discussed.

This lymphoma affects sinonasal tract and palate far more frequently than other types of non-Hodgkin's lymphomas, unlike in nasopharynx. Nasal natural killer (NK/T cell) lymphoma is an aggressive subtype of NHL, usually with a broad morphological spectrum, angioinvasion with necrosis, and is closely associated with Epstein Barr virus (EBV) infection (33). NK/T cell lymphoma is typically an extra nodal lymphoma with involvement of the gastrointestinal tract, skin, nasal cavities and pharynx. It was originally categorized as NK/T cell nasal lymphoma and those at other sites as NK/T cell non-nasal lymphoma. Now they are clubbed under the rubric extra nodal NK/T cell lymphoma (34). The most common presentation is with a destructive nasal or midline facial tumor, the so-called midline lethal granuloma.

Histologically, NK/T cell nasal lymphoma may show broad cytological spectrum but morphologically atypical cells are always present. These may vary from small and medium sized cells to large coarsely hyperchromatic pleomorphic cells (Figure 31 A, B). A prominent inflammatory infiltrate of plasma cells, histiocytes and eosinophils may obscure the tumors cells. The tumor is characteristically angiocentric and tumor cells infiltrate the vessel wall. A zonal pattern of necrosis is usually present, as sequelae of vascular compromise. Angiocentricity is defined as the presence of tumor cells around and within vascular lumina with infiltration and destruction of the vessel wall. Immunohistochemistry is necessary to confirm the cell type of this lymphoma. The tumor cells express T cell markers CD3 and CD 43, and typically CD56 positivity (Figure 31 C to E). Few cases of NK/T cell lymphoma are CD56 negative, in which case presence of T cell makers and EBV positivity confirm the diagnosis. Immunohistochemistry for EBER (EBV virus encoded RNA) is positive in over 95% of cases of NK/T cell lymphoma (35, 36).

Lymphomatoid granulomatosis, described below, shares many features of NK/T cell lymphoma and IHC is required for differentiation between the two.

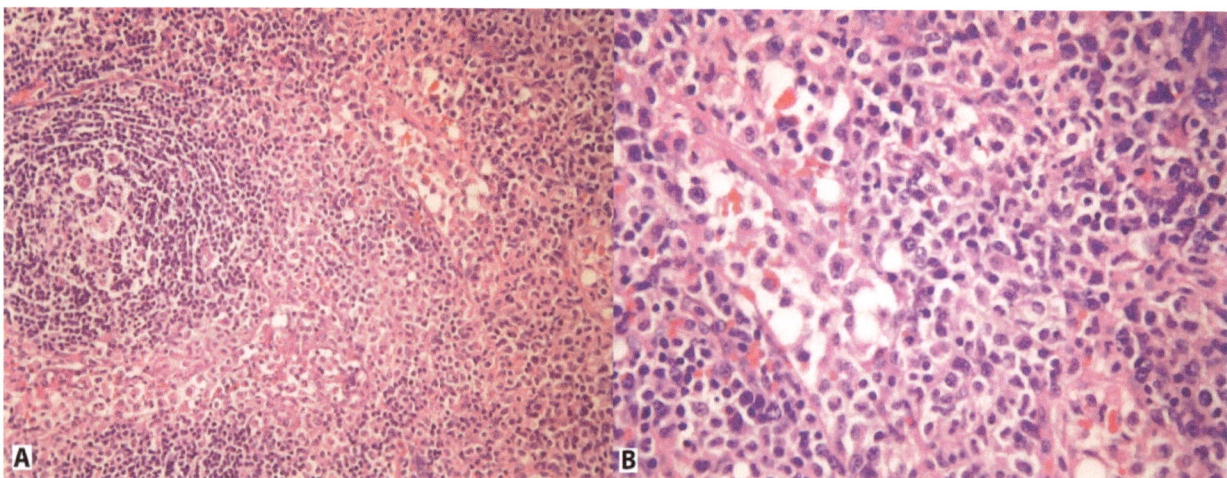

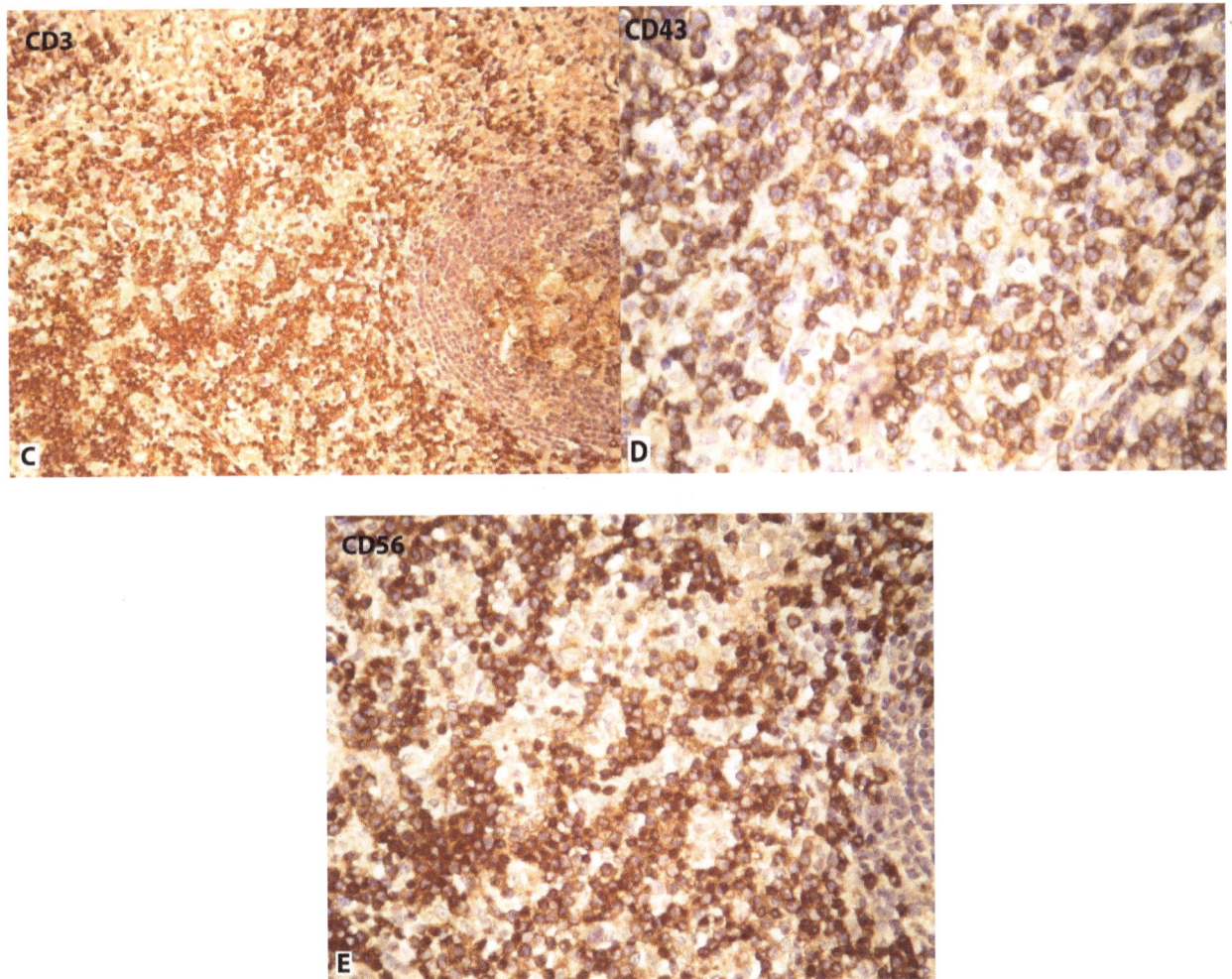

Figure 31 Maxillary N/KT lymphoma (A) diffuse large lymphocytes population with few inflammatory cells and one partly intact follicle; (B) very pleomorphic neoplastic lymphoid cells

Sjogren's syndrome (SS)

Definition and Clinical findings

Of the major autoimmune connective tissue diseases, Sjogren's syndrome (SS) is perhaps least understood. Both primary and secondary forms of SS occur but their phenotypes are not well defined. Primary Sjogren's syndrome (pSS) is an inflammatory autoimmune disease (Figure 32 (A, B) that predominantly affects salivary and lacrimal glands leading to progressive destruction of the glands and frequently accompanied by systemic symptoms. Involvement of non-exocrine organs including the lungs, kidney, thyroid and CNS has been reported in cases of pSS. In a large series of patients with pSS followed over 10 years, 33% were diagnosed to have one additional autoimmune disease, 6% had two and 2% had three. 51% of diagnoses of other autoimmune diseases were made before the diagnosis of pSS and 43% after the diagnosis of pSS. Although pSS remains a relatively benign disease, there is an increased tendency of developing additional autoimmune diseases. The secondary Sjogren's syndrome (SS) is defined as a patient with a well defined connective tissue disease and symptoms of ocular and oral dryness.

The patients with pSS may develop primary biliary cirrhosis, Sclerosing Cholangitis, pancreatitis, interstitial nephritis, interstitial lymphocytic pneumonia and peripheral vasculitis. The San Diego criteria for pSS include: keratoconjunctivitis sicca, xerostomia, extensive lymphocytic infiltrate on minor salivary gland biopsy, and laboratory evidence of systemic autoimmune disease. Histological study of minor or major salivary gland often reveals lymphoepithelial sialadenitis (also known as benign lymphoepithelial lesion, (Figure 32 C, D). This is characterized by heavy infiltration of marginal zone or monocytoid B cell lymphocytes in the ductal epithelium. In some cases, the lymphoepithelial lesion may have to be differentiated from lymphoepithelial carcinoma of nasopharyngeal type (37).

For a minor salivary gland biopsy diagnosis of SS, the specimen should include at least four salivary lobules with at least two foci of lymphocytic aggregates of 50 or more lymphocytes. Several sets of criteria for the diagnosis of SS have been proposed but the American-European (US-Eu) classification has been most commonly employed. No single test can serve as a gold standard but histopathology of the labial salivary gland remains a key feature in the sets of criteria. It should be noted that the labial biopsy resulted in 6%-9% false positive diagnoses and 18%-40% cases of clinically diagnosed SS had negative labial biopsy. Thus, the sensitivity of this test was found to be 60% to 82% and specificity 91% to 94%. The other disadvantages of labial biopsy are some degree of morbidity, inadequacy of salivary lobules in case of submucous atrophy and permanent sensory loss in 1%-10% of cases (38).

Some studies have shown that results of parotid gland biopsy are comparable with that of a labial biopsy and parotid biopsy may overcome some disadvantages of labial biopsy. Parotid tissue can be harvested easily and repeated biopsies are possible. In contrast to labial salivary glands, the diagnostic lymphoepithelial islands or lymphoepithelial lesions are often observed in parotid gland tissue of SS patients.

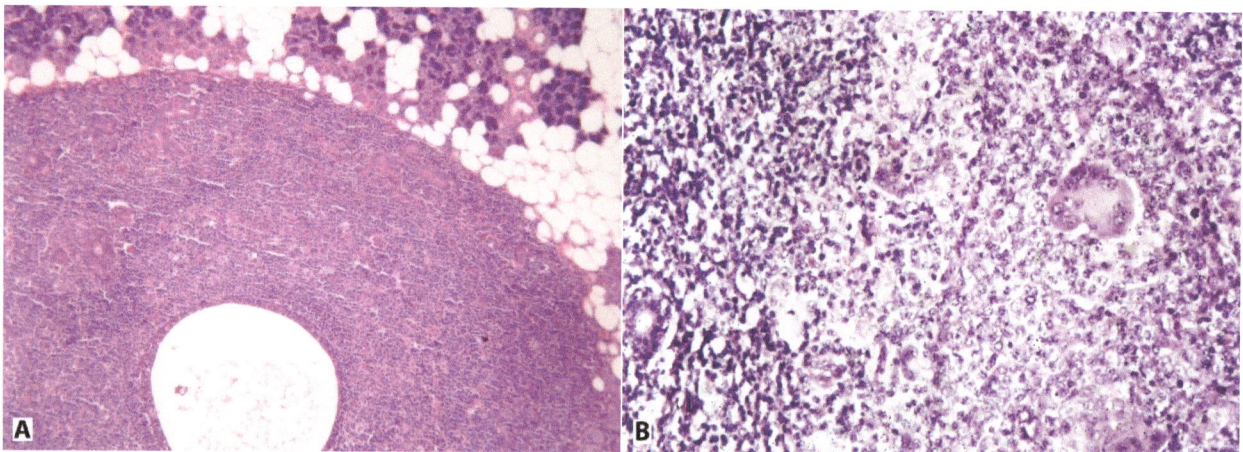

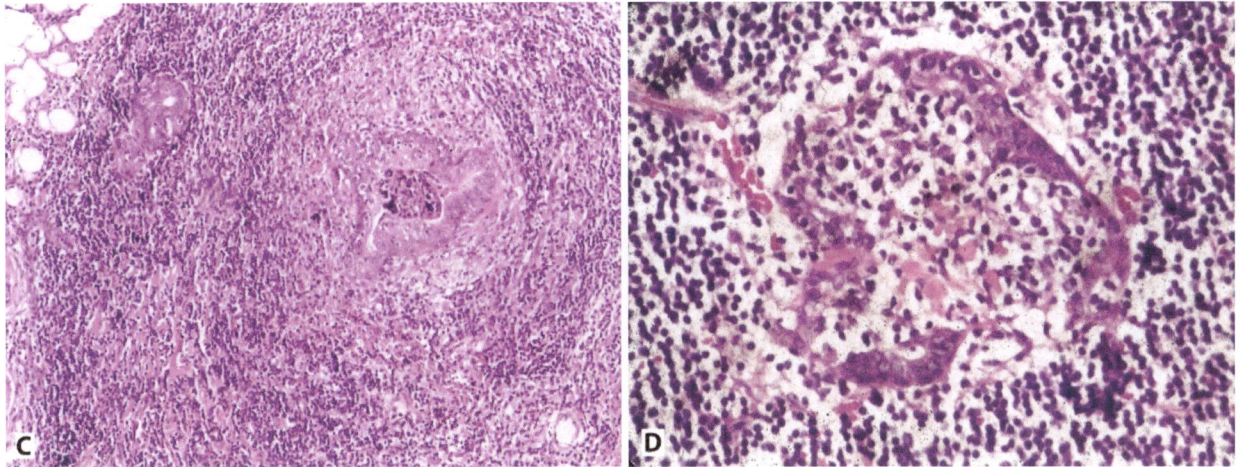

Figure 32 (A) A concentric lymphoid infiltrate around partly damaged parotid duct, (B) note multinucleated giant cell, (C & D) lymphoepithelial lesion

Lymphoma and Sjogren's syndrome

The occurrence of B cell non-Hodgkin lymphoma is a major complication in the evolution of SS, both in primary and secondary forms. In patients with SS followed over a period of over 15 years, NHL developed in 10%-15% of cases. NHL complicating SS arise not only in salivary glands but also in extra-nodal mucosal sites like lung and stomach. Most of these lymphomas are low grade MALT lymphomas (extranodal marginal B cell lymphoma). However, a small subset of these lymphomas evolves in to a high grade large B cell lymphoma (39) .

There are reports of association of hepatitis C virus (HCV) infection and SS. It is known that pSS is common in patients with primary biliary cirrhosis (PBC). More specifically, prevalence of autoimmune hepatitis in patients with pSS has been reported to be anywhere from 4% to a staggering high 47%. In one study on relation of HCV infection and SS, 19% of cases had anti-HCV antibodies in serum while only 10% of the patients had HCV viraemia. The histological study of salivary gland biopsy showed nodular lymphocytic infiltrates similar to that in pSS. In another study, 57% prevalence of focal lymphocytic sialadenitis suggestive of SS was found in 28 patients with chronic hepatitis C. In conclusion HCV infected patients could develop clinical and immunohistochemical patterns of salivary gland disease similar to that in pSS patients.

Lymphomatoid granulomatosis

Lymphomatoid granulomatosis, shares many features of NK/T cell lymphoma and IHC is required for differentiation between the two.

Definition and clinical findings

Lymphomatoid granulomatosis {LYG} represents a rare angiocentric and angiodestructive, EBV driven, T cell rich B cell lymphoproliferative disorder with clinical presentation varying from an indolent process to an aggressive B cell lymphoma. It is often associated with immunosuppression or immunodeficiency states and upper respiratory tract (20%), lung, oral cavity (40), CNS and skin are the most frequent sites of involvement. The designation lymphomatoid granulomatosis is incorrect because the lesion is not granulomatous morphologically. The zones of necrosis are bordered by lymphocytes and not histiocytes, unlike in mycobacterial or fungal infections.

The histopathology varies according to the grade of the disease. Initially (Grade I) the pattern is of extensive CD4 positive lymphocytic infiltration of the vessel wall with no apparent vascular injury, and lymphocytes with only a few EBV infected B cells (less than 5 EBV affected B cells per high power field); reactive CD8 lymphocytes are very few in number. The T cells may show atypia and T cell clonality may occur. In the next stage there is fibrinoid necrosis of the vessel wall with variable luminal thrombosis (Grade II). At this stage EBV positive B cell population increases progressively (5–20 EBV infected cells per high power field) and in grade III cases sheet like growth of EBV positive cells is indicative of transformation of the lesion into diffuse large B cell lymphoma.

It is important to know that in NK/T cell lymphoma EBV is detected in CD4 lymphocytes, whereas in LYG EBV is localized in B lymphocytes. LYG is thus an immunodysregulatory disorder of B and T lymphocytes and further evolution develops into a B cell lymphoma after a variable interval. About one third of grade 1 and two-thirds of grade 2 lesions progress to lymphoma (41). Vascular patterns of LYG assume two morphologic variations. The first and most common is characterized by extensive infiltration of the vessel by CD4 positive lymphocytes unaccompanied by vessel wall injury. The second pattern is one characterized by fibrinoid necrosis of the vessel wall with variable intraluminal thrombosis. The vascular damage may be mediated by the chemokines IP-10 and Mig, which are overexpressed in involved tissues (42a).

LYG was first described in 1972 by Liebow as a new disease occurring in lung that shared overlapping features with lymphoma and Wegner's granulomatosis (42). The most common radiographic picture is the presence of multiple rounded mass densities that are bilateral and mainly in the lower lobes. Clinically and radiologically the disease resembles WG but biopsy findings are more suggestive of lymphoma. This topic will be discussed in detail and illustrated in Chapter on neoplasms of Lung.

Lesions of Sinonasal Tract mimicking tumors

Table 8: Lesions of Sinonasal tract (n = 2855) Author's series (1970-2005)	
Inflammatory and Non contributory	341
Specific Infections & Granulomas	486
Polyps	981
Papillomas	177
Miscellaneous benign**	330
Skin lesions	60
Malignant tumors	480

** Cysts, teratomas, tumors of soft tissues & bones

Nose is the first barrier to infective or toxic products inhaled from the environment and consequently a variety of bacterial and fungal infection occur in this organ. Majority of these infections (Table 9) are readily identified. A few of these, however, can be overlooked or totally missed. A few present as a mass lesion, which may be clinically indistinguishable from a neoplasm and pertinent cases are illustrated (Figure 33, 34, 35).

Table 9: Special Infective & other granulomatous Lesions of sinonasal tract (n =492) Author's series	
Rhinoscleroma	223
Rhinosporiodiosis	137
Mucormycosis	32
Aspergillosis	20
Enteromopthoramycosis	8
Actinomycosis/Nocardia	2
Fungal infection (NOS)	9
Leishmaniasis	1
Tuberculosis	42
Hansen's disease	6
Granuloma (NOS)	6
Malakoplakia	1
Wegener's granulomatosis	5

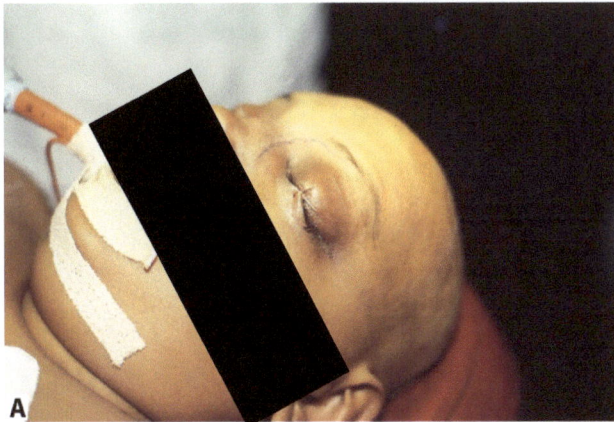

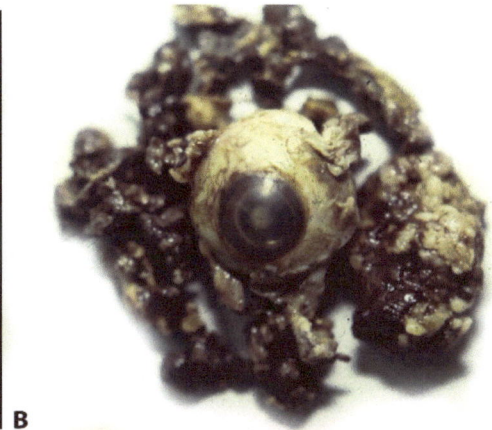

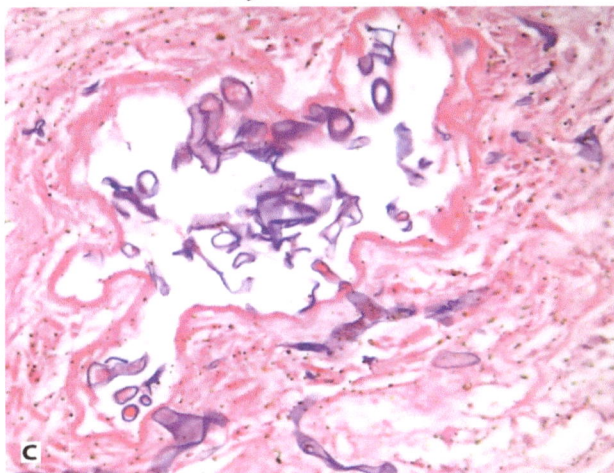

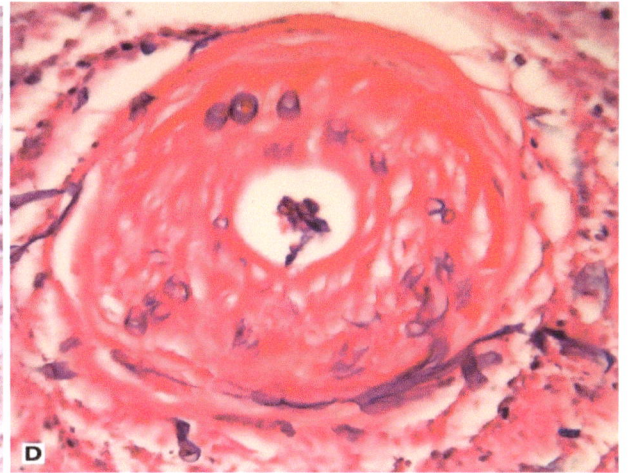

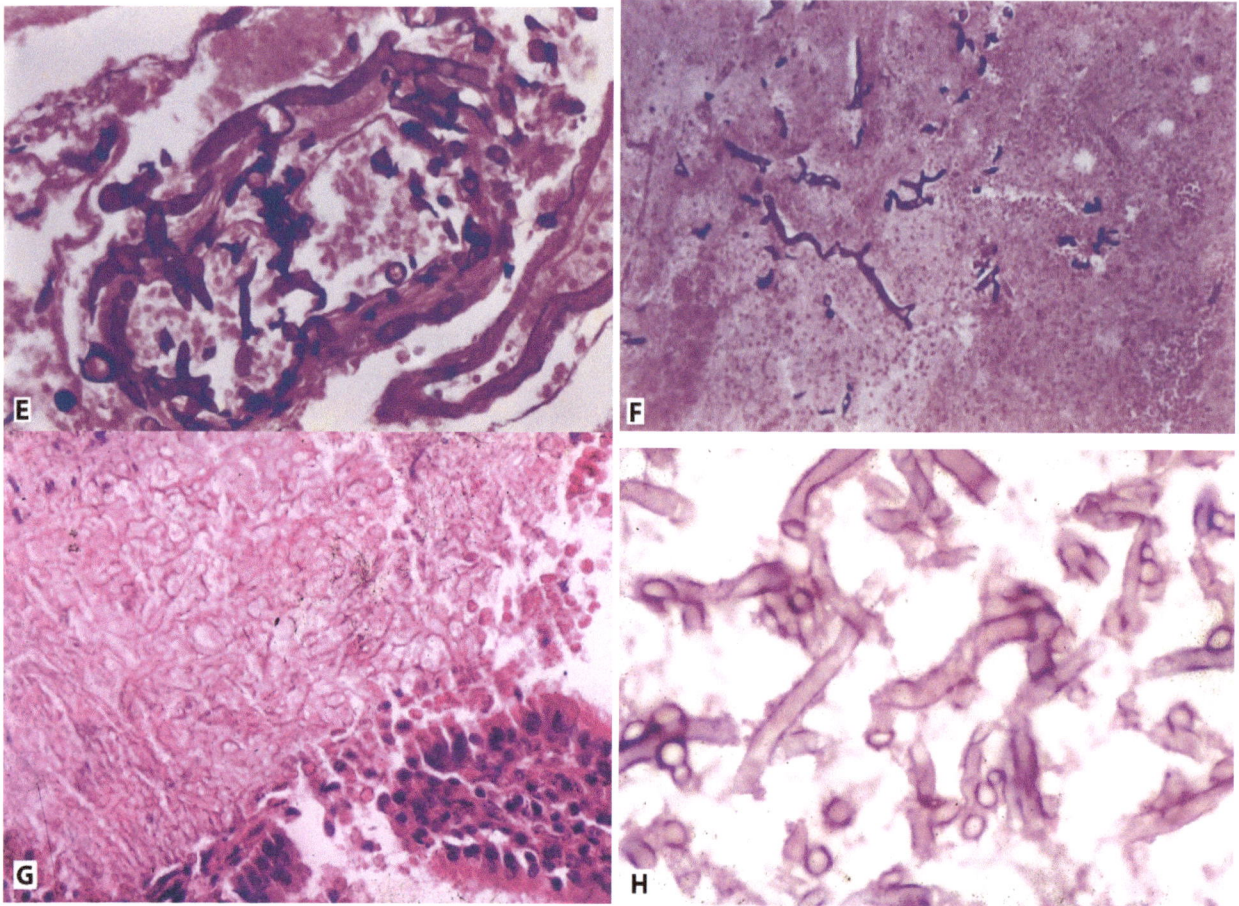

Figure 33 Mucor mycosis: (A) diffuse mass lesion in orbit, (B) ennucleated orbital contents (C & D) mucor hyphae, spores in soft tissues and a thick vessel, (E) mucor embolus in a vessel, (F) mucor hyphae in the cerebrum, (G, H) Nasal aspergillosis

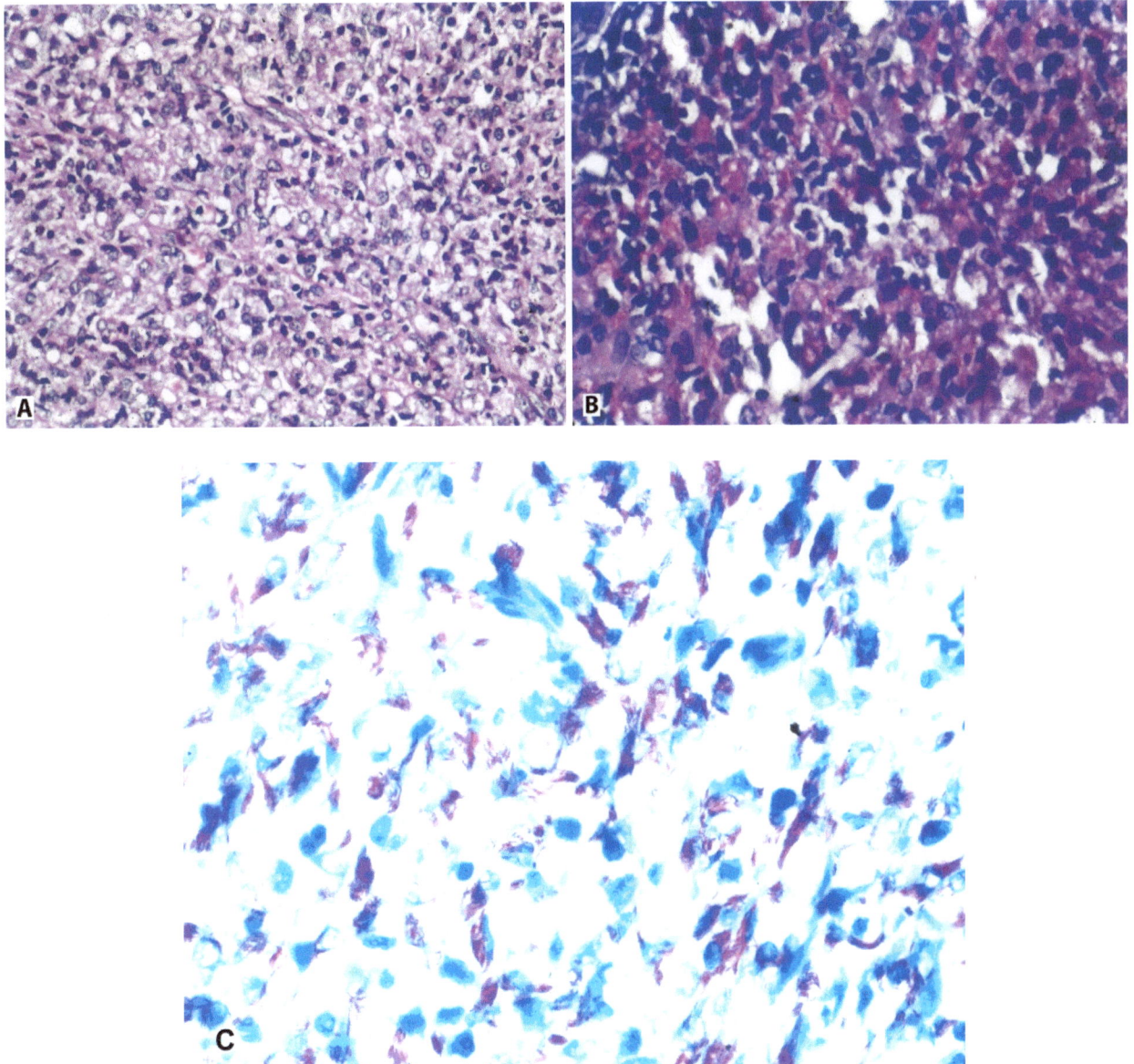

Figure 34 Hansen's disease: (A) mass lesion in the nose, biopsied nodule packed with histiocytes, (B) cells filled with lepra bacilli, H & E counterstained (C) ZN stain show clusters of lepra bacilli on a tissue section

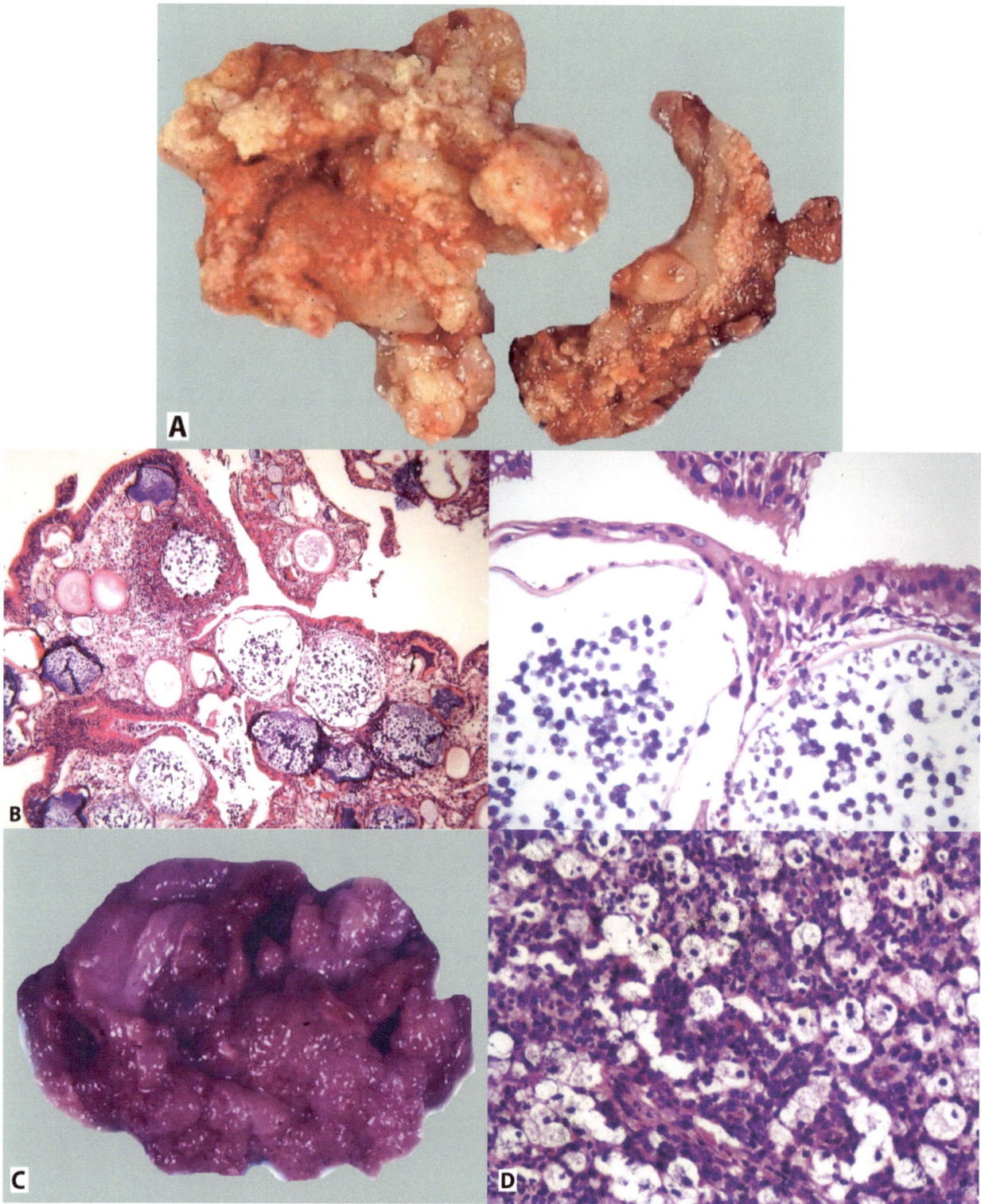

Figure 35 (A) polpoid nasal mass (B) rhinosporidia (C) this mass was clinically suspected to be a neoplasm; (D) vacuolated Mickulicz cells and plasma cells typical of rhinoscleroma

Table 10: Malignant Tumors of Sinonasal Tract (n = 480) Authors' s series (1970-2005)	
Squamous Cell Carcinoma*	167
Adenocarcinoma (NOS)	75
Adenoid cystic carcinoma	3
Small cell undifferentiated ("oat" cell) carcinoma	15
Papillary carcinoma	10
Lymphoepithelial carcinoma (nasopharyngeal type)**	7
Undifferentiated carcinoma	38
Total carcinomas	345
Olfactory Neuroblastoma	36
NHL	33
Plasma cell Myeloma	6
Soft Tissue Sarcomas	53

* refer to section on squamous cell carcinomas of aero digestive tract

** described in detail in the section on Lymphoproliferative disorders of Head & Neck

Carcinomas of Sinonasal Tract & Salivary glands

Small cell undifferentiated carcinomas express neuroendocrine markers: synaptophysin, chromogranin and NSE. Undifferentiated carcinomas are stained with epithelial markers and are negative for neuroendocrine markers. Among cases of adenocarcinoma, adenoid cystic carcinoma stands apart because of its high mortality despite innocuous (low grade) morphology and rather indolent growth. This will be described in brief.

Adenoid cystic carcinoma (ACC) is a basaloid tumor consisting of epithelial and myoepithelial cells in variable morphologic conFigureurations, including tubular, cribriform and solid patterns (Figure 36 A-D). Grossly, the tumor is unencapsulated and invariably infiltrative. The cribriform pattern, the most frequent, is characterized by nests of cells with cylindromatous microcystic spaces filled with hyaline or basophilic mucoid material. A pure solid histological form may be difficult to identify and

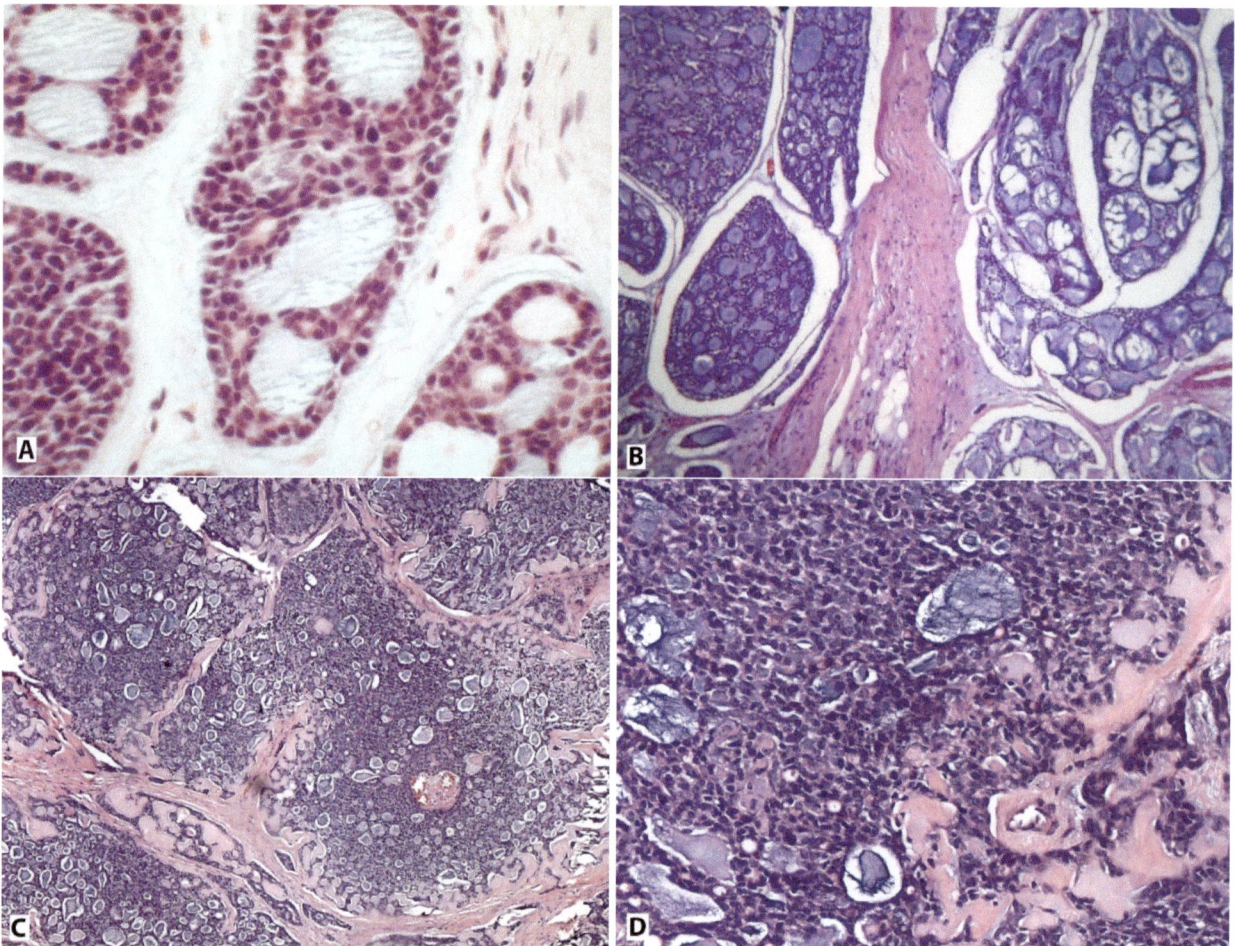

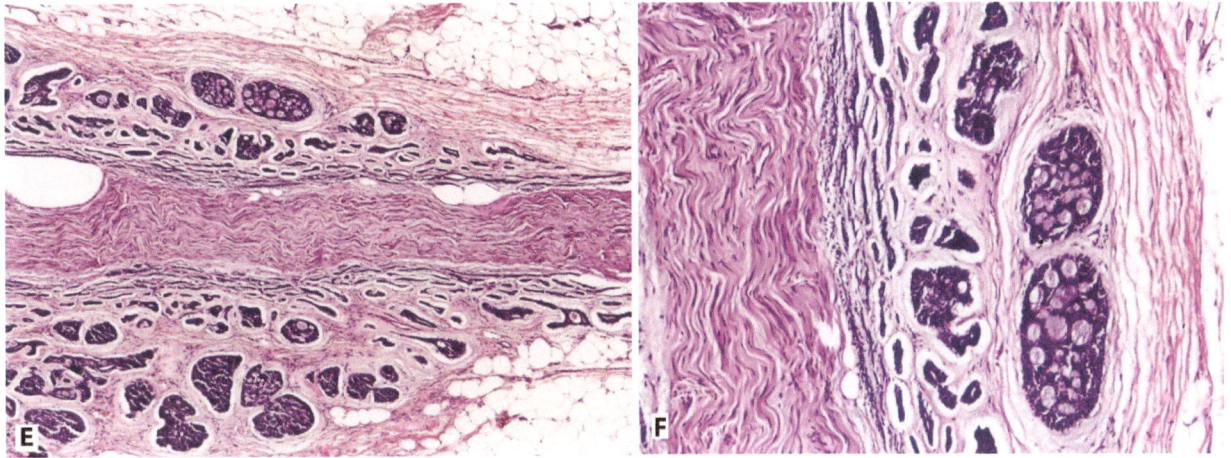

Figure 36 (A to D) various patterns of adenoid cystic carcinoma (E, F) extensive neural and perineural infiltration

differentiate from polymorphous low grade adenocarcinoma, basal cell adenoma or adenocarcinoma and basaloid squamous cell carcinoma on a small biopsy. The long term poor prognosis of ACC is due to its relentless spread along the nerves. Lymph nodal metastasis is very rare indeed.

In a large study of thirty articles yielded usable data on a total of 1065 patients with adenoid cystic carcinoma (43) for analysis: expected 5-year survival rate was 62.4% and 10-year survival rate was a poor 38.9%.

Sinonasal undifferentiated carcinoma:

(Synonym: Anaplastic carcinoma)

Squamous cell carcinoma, including keratinizing and nonkeratinizing types is the most commonly encountered malignant neoplasm of the sinonasal tract. From this small but complex anatomic region, a variety of clinically aggressive high-grade epithelial as well as nonepithelial malignant neoplasms arise with overlapping clinical and light microscopic features; making differentiation of one from the other difficult without the use of ancillary studies such as immunohistochemistry, electron microscopy, molecular biology. Differentiating these tumor types has a great clinical importance as advances in targeted therapeutic intervention per tumor type may increase survival, enhance quality of life, and occasionally result in a cure (43a).

Sinonasal undifferentiated carcinoma (SNUC) was first described in 1986 by Frierson et al. (43b). SNUC is a rare but extremely malignant neoplasm characterized by rapid growth, a propensity for loco regional recurrence, distant metastases particularly to lung and bone, and poor prognosis. Most reports cite poor outcomes regardless of treatment strategy. An aggressive multimodality approach including surgery, radiation, and chemotherapy offers the best chance for loco regional control and cure.

SNUC is believed to originate from Shneiderian epithelium or from the nasal ectoderm of the paranasal sinuses (43a). It is thought to be a member of the neuroendocrine group of sinonasal malignancies that also includes esthesioneuroblastoma, neuroendocrine carcinoma, and small cell carcinoma. However, in the current WHO classification (2005), it is listed under epithelial malignancy.

Histologically, SNUC is classically composed of small to medium-sized undifferentiated cells with high mitotic rates, marked nuclear pleomorphism, high nuclear to cytoplasmic ratios, inconspicuous to prominent nucleoli, extensive necrosis and apoptosis, extensive angiolymphatic invasion and no evidence of neuroendocrine differentiation (i.e. no Homer Wright rosettes, no fibrillary background, no ganglion-like cells). These tumors lack squamous or glandular differentiation. Immunohistochemical analysis is useful to confirm the diagnosis. The tumor cells are strongly positive for cytokeratin, particularly cytokeratin 7, 8, and 19 and negative for cytokeratin 5/6 and 13. SNUC are negative for EBV. In addition, they are often positive for neuron-specific enolase and chromogranin, have slight overlap with olfactory neuroblastoma and neuroendocrine carcinomas. SNUC is often nonreactive to S-100 and never expresses vimentin which is helpful in separating it from other neuroendocrine carcinomas.

Undifferentiated Nasopharyngeal carcinomas in contrast are cytokeratin 5/6 & 13 (high molecular weight cytokeratin) positive, EBV positive, rarely have vascular invasion and usually show little destruction or spread.

The histogenesis and classification of SNUC remain questionable and debatable, necessitating further studies on this tumor type to answer some of these open issues (43a, 43b).

Table 11: LESIONS OF SALIVARY GLANDS (N = 1701) Author's series (1970-2005)	
Non-contributory & Inflammatory	408 (23.98%)
Specific Non-neoplastic lesions	93 (05.47%)
Benign epithelial tumors	738 (43.40%)
Benign Non-epithelial tumors	31 (1.82%)
Cysts	52 (3.06%)
Malignant tumors	379 (22.28%)
Specific Non-neoplastic Lesions of Salivary glands	(N = 93)

Table 12: Specific Non-neoplastic Lesions of Salivary glands (N = 93) (Mass forming lesions) Author's series (1970-2005)	
Tuberculosis	70
Sarcoidosis	11
Sjogren's **	12

Malignant Tumors of Salivary Glands

Benign mixed tumor or pleomorphic adenoma is the most common tumor of both major and minor salivary glands accounting for 40% to 70% of all neoplasms of these organs. In our experience of 1117 salivary gland tumors 52% were pleomorphic adenomas. Malignant tumors are relatively uncommon individually but collectively the volume is large enough, requiring special attention and expertise in diagnosis and classification. The difficulties in the interpretation of malignant salivary tumors arise as a result of broad histological spectrum with significant morphological overlap. A fair number of these tumors do not easily fit into existing diagnostic categories and establishing histologically malignant nature of some of these indolent low grade neoplasms is difficult.

Table 13: Malignant Tumors of Salivary glands (N = 379) Author's series (1970-2005)	
Mucoepidermoid carcinoma	123 (32.45%)
Adenoid cystic carcinoma	68 (17.94%)
Clear cell carcinoma	10 (2.64%)
Acinic cell carcinoma	8 (2.11%)
Mucinous carcinoma	3 (0.79%)
Adenocarcinoma NOS	33 (8.7%)
Basal cell adenocarcinoma	2 (0.52%)
Malignant mixed tumor	19 (5%)
Epithelial myoepithelial carcinoma	1 (0.26%)
Malignant myoepithelioma	1 (0.26%)
Squamous cell carcinoma	20 (5.27%)
Small cell undifferentiated carcinoma	44 (11.6%)
NHL	27 (7.12%)
Sarcoma	9 (2.37%)
Metastatic from other sites	11 (2.9%)

Mucoepidermoid carcinoma, adenoid cystic carcinoma, clear cell carcinoma, acinic cell carcinoma and mucinous adenocarcinoma are all morphologically distinct and easily diagnosed. There are noteworthy differences in the biological behavior and prognosis of these tumors. There is a pool of adenocarcinoma which has been designated as adenocarcinoma not otherwise specified (NOS) and over the last 15 years or so newer morphological entities have been separated from adenocarcinoma NOS group. These include polymorphous low grade adenocarcinoma, salivary duct carcinoma, basal cell adenocarcinoma, malignant sebaceous tumor, oncocytic carcinoma and cystadenocarcinoma.

Malignant mixed tumors of salivary gland will be discussed along with myoepithelial carcinoma and epithelial-myoepithelial carcinoma. The latter two neoplasms in our own series were lumped with malignant mixed tumors, in the past. Myoepithelial carcinoma and epithelial-myoepithelial carcinoma have been selected particularly because they are rare, often simulate each other, have different biological behavior and need a battery of immunostains for accurate classification.

Polymorphous low grade adenocarcinoma

A rare, low grade, infiltrative, morphologically diverse, adenocarcinoma has a low malignant potential. Nearly 60% occur in the palate and the less common sites in the descending order are buccal mucosa, base of tongue and major salivary glands. The tumor cells are medium sized cuboidal and strikingly uniform small vesicular nuclei. There is hardly any mitotic activity (44). The tumor exhibits a variety of patterns, namely; papillary, trabecular, lobular and rarely cribriform (like in adenoid cystic carcinoma) (Figure 37. The differentiation from other adenocarcinoma may be difficult if the biopsy is small.

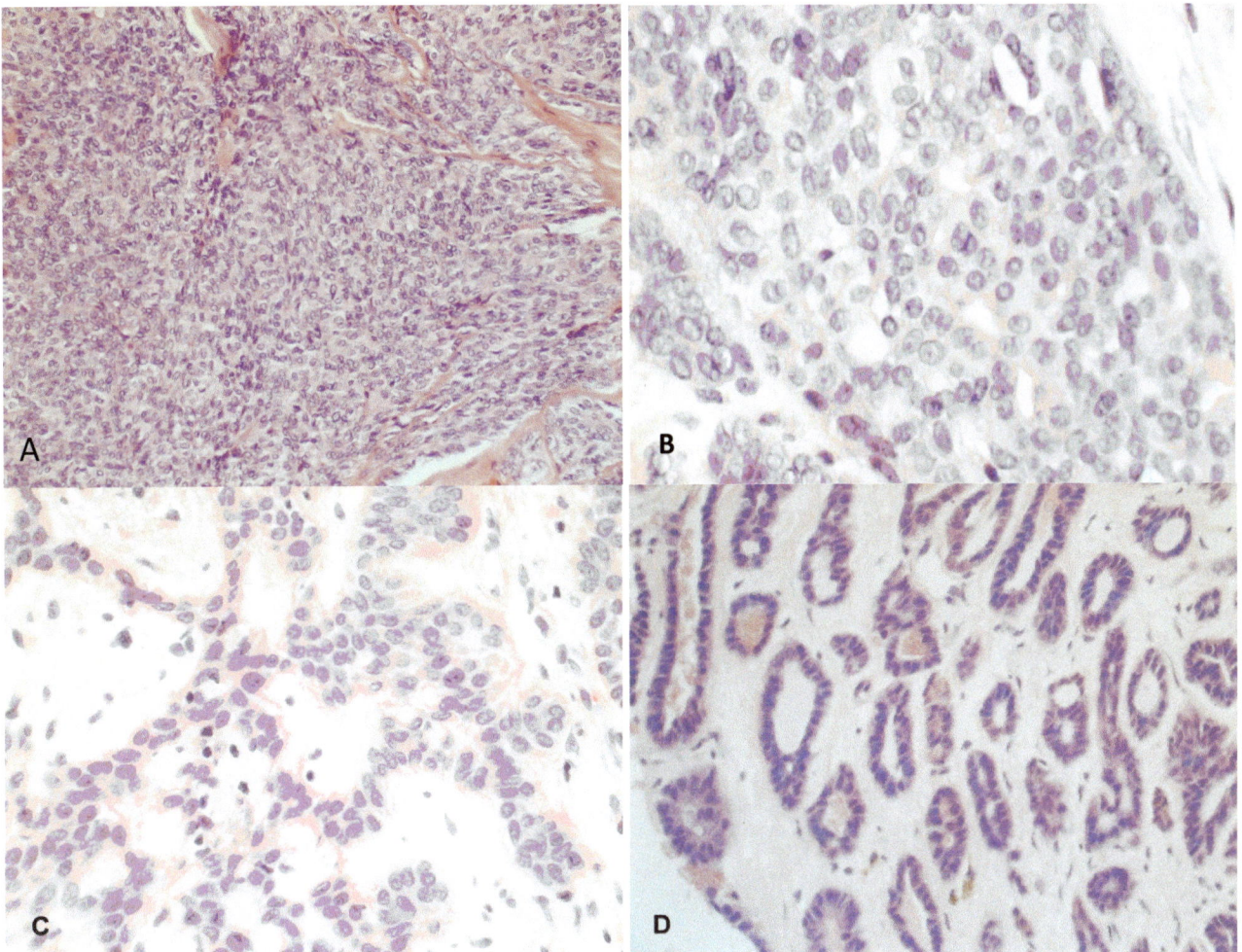

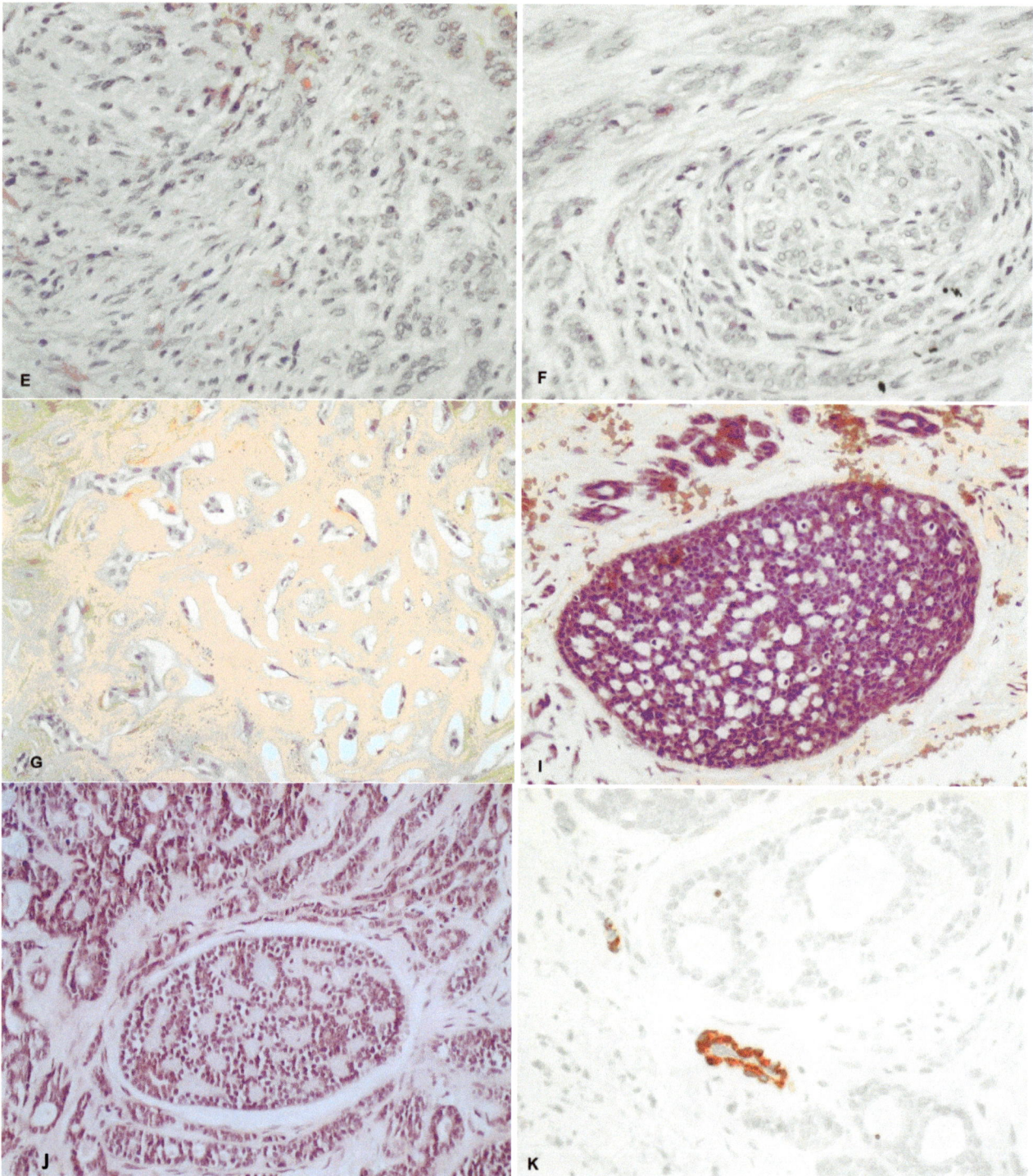

(Figure 37) (A,B) PLGA with solid pattern, (C,D) PLGA with tubular pattern; (E,F) PLGA with perineural invasion; (G) PLGA with areas of hyalinization; (I,J) PLGA with adenoid cystic carcinoma pattern; (K) Smooth Muscle Myosin Heavy Chain (SMMHC) highlighting lack of myoepithelial lining

Salivary duct carcinoma

(Figure 38 A)

This is a rare variety of salivary adenocarcinoma with a striking resemblance to high grade ductal carcinoma of breast with comedo necrosis and high mortality rate. The tumor cells are large with abundant cytoplasm and large actively mitotic pleomorphic nuclei. The cells display intraductal with infiltrating duct pattern with central necrosis in tumor islands. It is quite aggressive with high incidence of perineural invasion, nearly 60% lymph node metastasis and frequent blood borne metastases. Clinically, the tumors are characterized by aggressive behavior with early nodal metastasis, local recurrence and significant mortality (45).

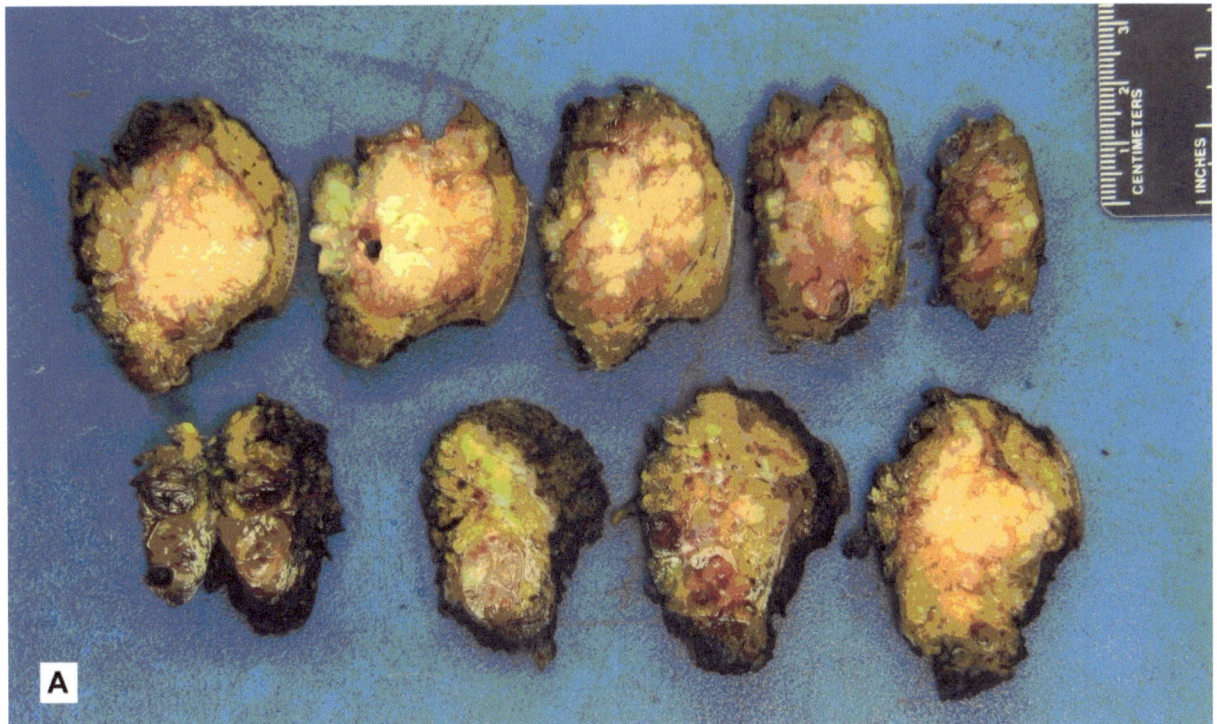

A

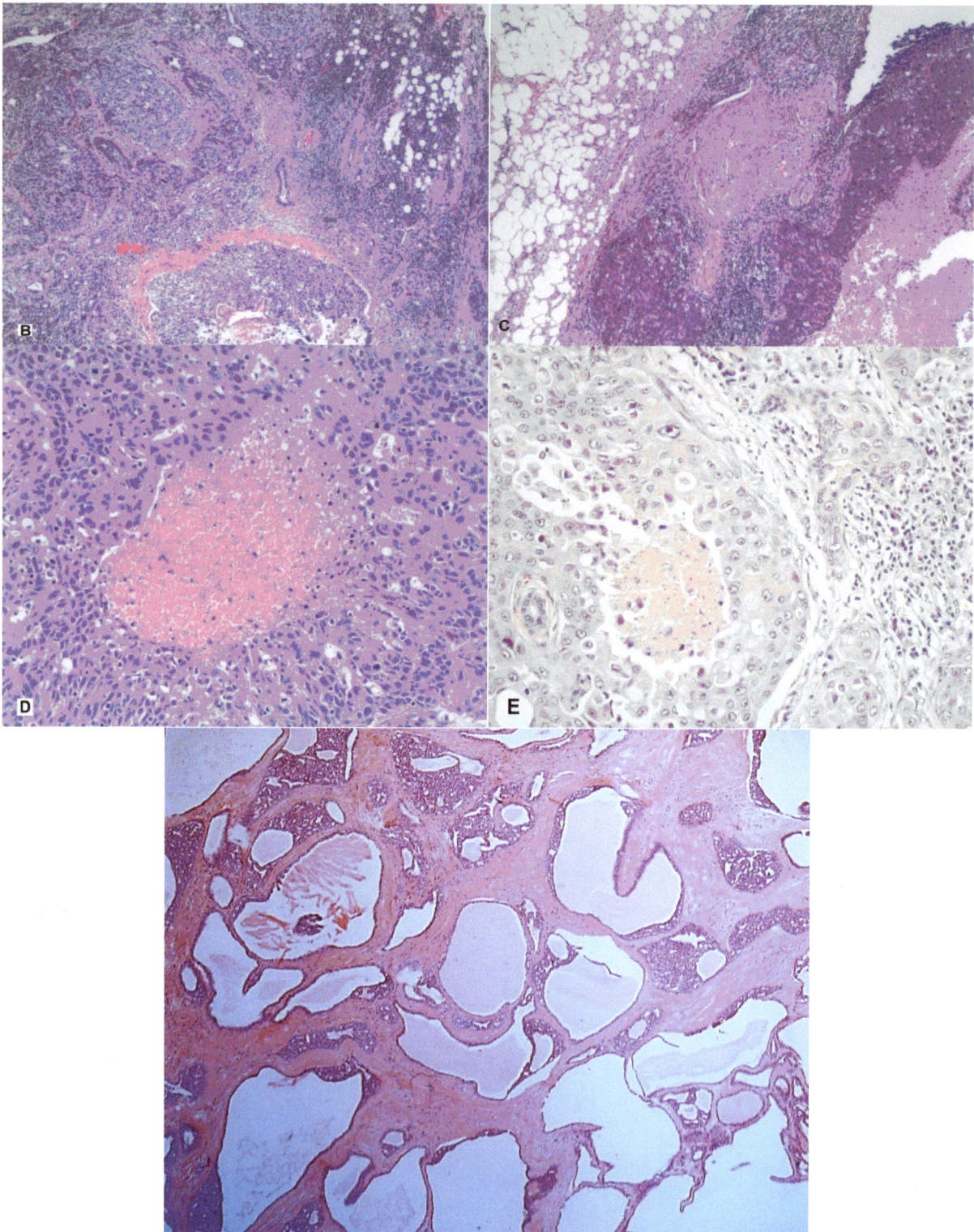

Figure 38 (A) Gross photograph of ductal salivary gland adenocarcinoma (B,C) H&E Low Power microscopic features of ductal salivary gland adenocarcinoma; (D,E) High power showing comedonecrosis (F) Low grade salivary duct carcinoma mimicking cystadenoma

High grade transformation in adenocarcinoma of salivary gland

Transformation of an adenocarcinoma into anaplastic or dedifferentiated form is not uncommon and has been reported in adenoid cystic carcinoma, acinic cell adenocarcinoma, polymorphous low grade adenocarcinoma etc (46). One may argue about the terminology analogous to chondrosarcoma, where such morphologic change has been categorized as "de-differentiation". One example, that of dedifferentiated adenoid cystic carcinoma (Figure 39 A, B), is illustrated below. It is stressed that in such cases immunohistochemistry is quite helpful for an accurate histogenetic diagnosis (Figure 39 C, D).

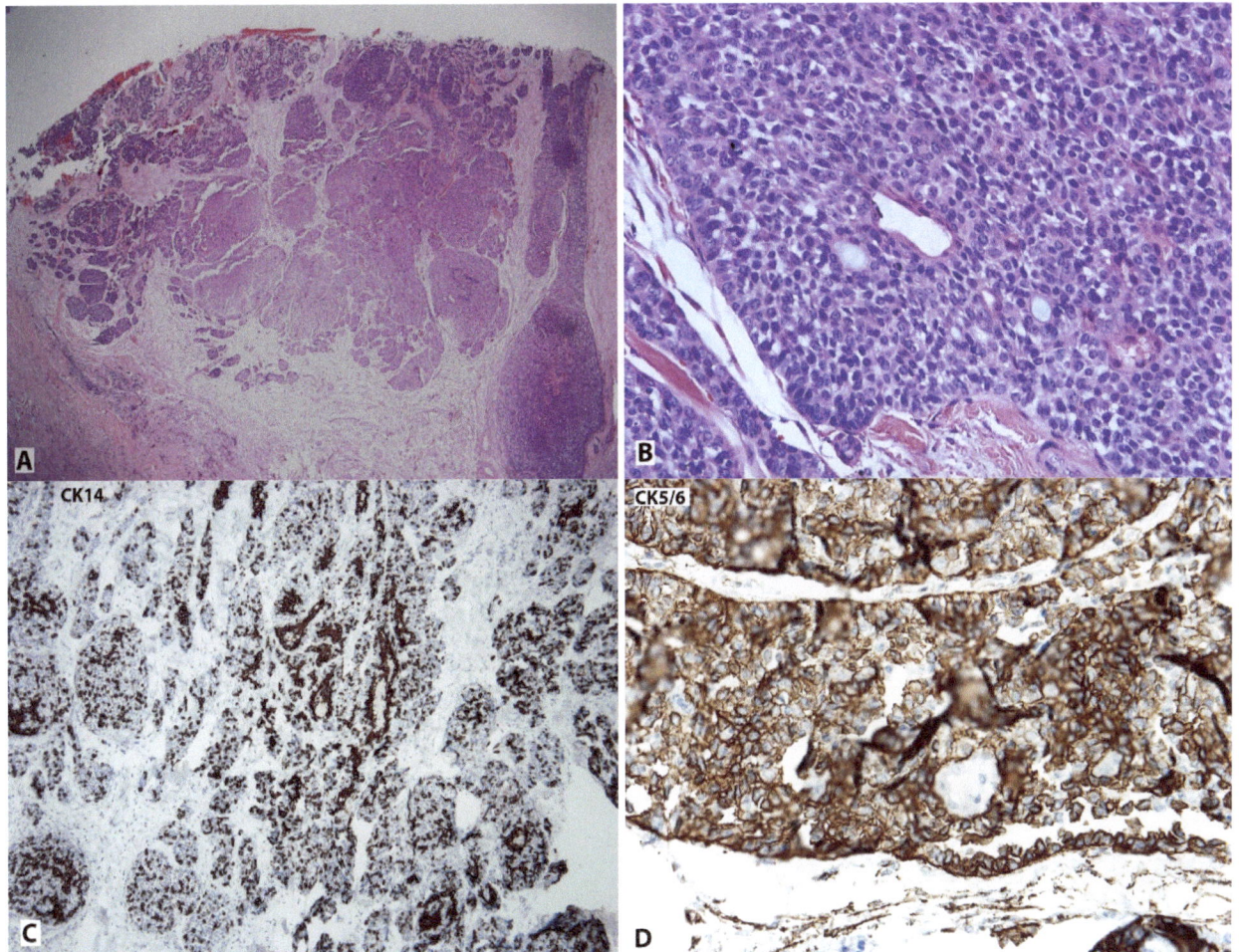

Figure 39 (A&B) dedifferentiated adenoid cystic carcinoma (C) high molecular weight keratin (CK14) for luminal cells (D) myoepithelial cells express (CK 5/6)

Myoepithelial Carcinoma

(Figure 40 A-H)

Myoepithelioma is a rare tumor of myoepithelial cells that was recognized as a distinct entity by the WHO in 1991. It is accepted that pleomorphic adenoma and myoepithelioma represent a morphological spectrum with lesions dominated by ductal structures, myxoid stroma and only few myoepithelial cells at one end and neoplasm composed purely of myoepithelial cells at the other end.

Myoepithelial carcinoma (MC) is a malignant counterpart of myoepithelioma and in the past it was lumped with malignant mixed tumor. As of 1985 only 3 cases were found in the literature and the tally was 75 cases by the year 2002. Its proper delineation evolved in the next 10 years and detailed histology of all varied morphologic patterns was described. The tumor presents, multinodularity with a cellular periphery, central necrotic or myxoid tissue, and lack of encapsulation. The neoplastic myoepithelial cells present a variety of forms, namely: epithelioid, spindly, plasmacytoid, hyaline, clear cell and mixed types. Mixed cell population with two or more cell types is a most commonly encountered pattern. The fundamental histologic criteria of myoepithelial carcinoma are exclusively myoepithelial cell population and unequivocal evidence of malignancy in the tumor. A battery of immunohistochemical tests is necessary to confirm the diagnosis and differentiating it from many other types of salivary tumors. In one large study imunoreactivity included AE1:AE 3 (100%), 34BE12 (100%) as epithelial markers and vimentin (100%), S100 (100%) and calponin (75%) as myoepithelial markers. Few reports in the literature refer to predominantly myoepithelial cells with some luminal cell (tubular) differentiation. Consensus among the experts is that the designation myoepithelial carcinoma should be reserved for cases with exclusive myoepithelial differentiation. Cases with focal tubular differentiation should be classified as epithelial myoepithelial carcinoma (47).

Assessment of malignancy in myoepithelial tumor is not all that easy. The traditional criteria for discriminating benign and malignant myoepithelioma include cytologic atypia, tumor infiltration and mitotic activity. However, these fail to predict the clinical outcome. It has been suggested that Ki 67 index of more than 10% is diagnostic of myoepithelial carcinoma. The clinical behavior and outcome of myoepithelial carcinoma is remarkably variable so that cases showing aggressive histological features have remained indolent and lived as long as 8 to 15 years post treatment. Occasionally, low grade tumors with minimal mitotic activity have metastasized. In general, pleomorphism, coarse chromatin, prominent nucleoli, mitotic Figures and necrosis are observed in obviously malignant myoepithelial carcinoma. Such cases will need a more aggressive surgical approach (48).

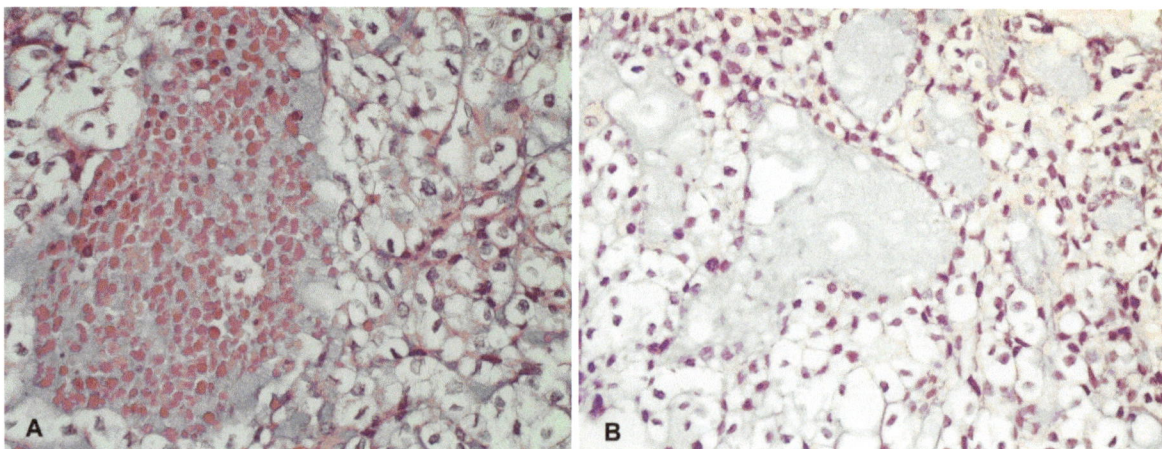

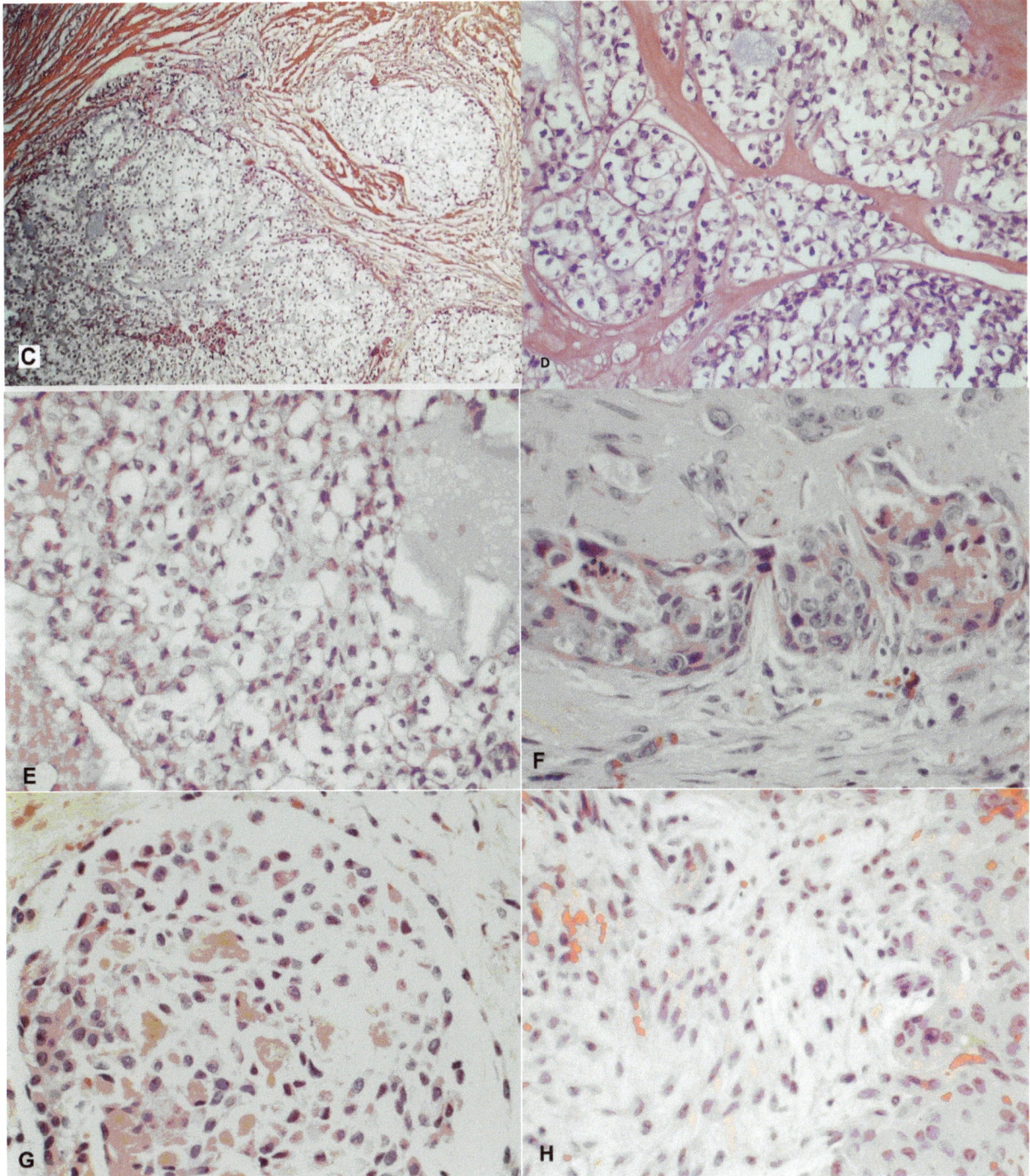

Figure 40 (A) MC with foci of necrosis; (B) MC with myxoid areas; (C) MC with lobular pattern; (D) MC with clear cells and stromal hyalinization; (E) MC with clear cell areas; (F) MC with high nuclear grade; (G,H) MC with plasmacytoid features

Epithelial Myoepithelial Carcinoma

This is a malignant tumor composed of ductal structures lined by a single layer of ductal cells {epithelial} surrounded by single or multiple layers of clear myoepithelial cells. It is a relatively low grade malignancy and recurrence is reported in 30% to 40% of cases, which may occur as late as 28 years after initial surgery (49). Regional lymph node metastases occur in 10% to 20% but a case with distant metastasis is rather uncommon.

The ductal cells are strongly positive for pan cytokeratin and variably positive for S100 protein but are negative for myoepithelial markers. Markers of myoepithelium include p53, actin and calponin. The proliferation index is low: 1% for ductal cells and <3% for abluminal cells (50).

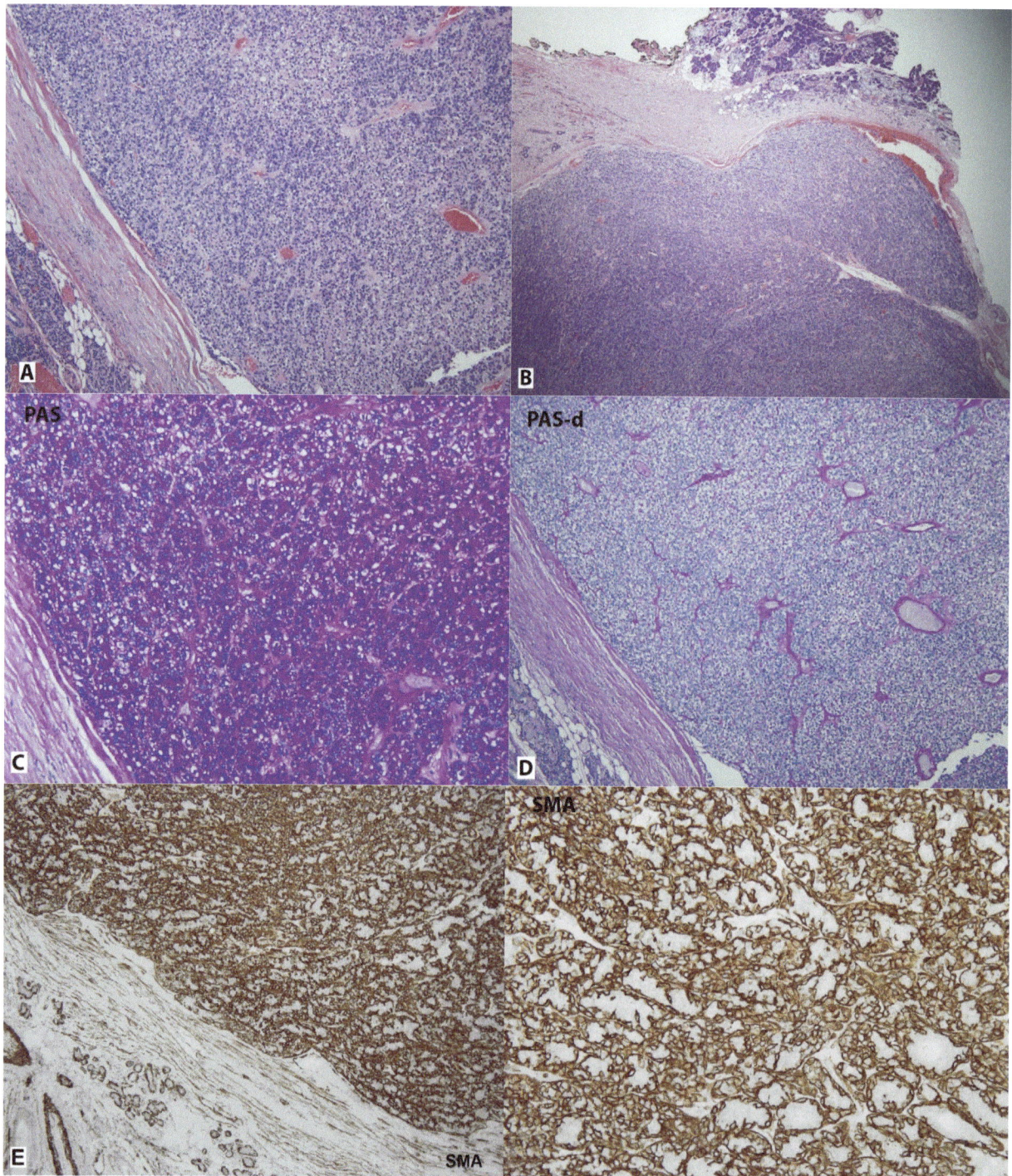

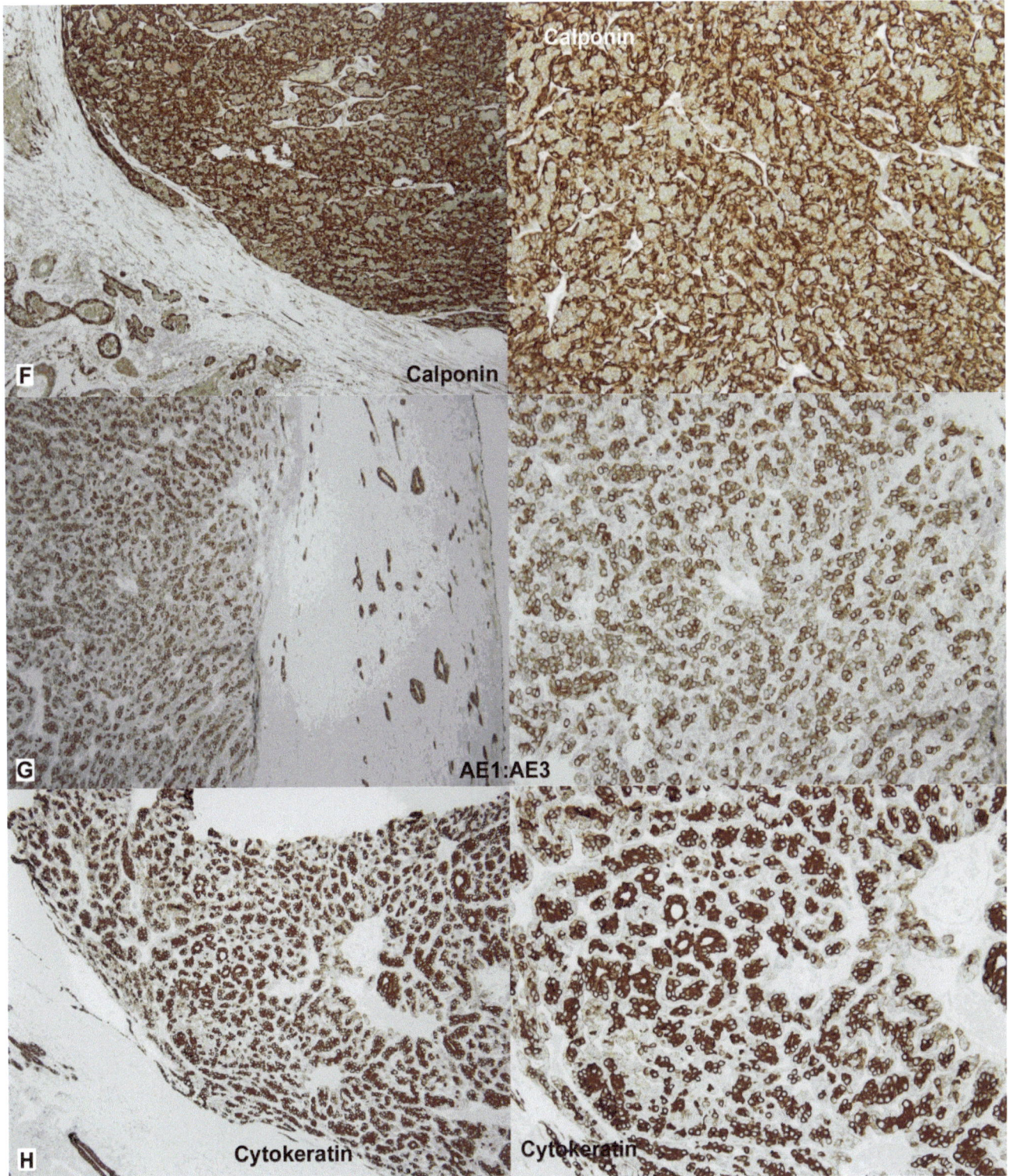

Figure 41 (A,B) Scanner veiw of epithelial – myoepithelial carcinoma; (C,D) clear cell pattern due to cytoplasmic glycogen (stained with PAS – Diastase); (E,F) SMA and calponin highlighting myoepithelial cells; (G,H) AE1:AE3 and cytokeratin for ductal columnar epithelial cells.

Hybrid carcinoma

There are a few articles which have reported a "distinct entity" called hybrid carcinoma of salivary glands (48). It is characterized by a combination of two distinct histological types of tumor within the same topographical areas. The concept of hybrid carcinoma is subject to certain degree of confusion. Malignant mixed tumors, far instance, are not regarded as Hybrid tumors. It is clear that hybrid carcinomas are composed of two different malignant epithelial tumor elements. Various carcinoma combinations have been described in hybrid carcinomas; salivary duct carcinoma, epithelial myoepithelial carcinoma and adenoid cystic carcinoma are frequently involved. Less commonly basal cell adenocarcinoma, squamous cell carcinoma, myoepithelial carcinoma etc form part of the combination. Not all tumors with two or more morphologies are considered hybrid tumors. Thus entities like collision tumors, synchronous/metachronous tumors, dedifferentiated carcinoma, sarcomatoid carcinoma and adenosquamous carcinoma are not considered hybrid carcinomas. The type of treatment and prognosis are related to the more aggressive high grade tumor component in the combination.

The authors believe that there is no need of creating an entity with a label hybrid carcinoma. It is unnecessarily confusing and serves no useful function. Tumors exhibiting different histological subtypes should be documented with detailed histological features and graded and staged by the usual criteria. The component with higher grade morphology will determine the type of treatment and assess prognosis.

Malignant mixed tumors

Malignant mixed tumor (MMT), is a counterpart of the frequently encountered benign mixed tumor of salivary tissues. The designation malignant mixed tumor is employed, when remnants of benign mixed tumor are identified within a tumor composed of malignant epithelial and mesenchymal cells. It is indeed rare. Within the broad heading of "malignant mixed tumor are included three different entities (51):

1) True malignant mixed tumor (carcinosarcoma)

2) Carcinoma arising in a mixed tumor (Carcinoma ex mixed tumor)

3) Metastasizing benign mixed tumor.

True Malignant Mixed Tumor (Carcinosarcoma)

True malignant mixed tumor or carcinosarcoma arises in a preexisting pleomorphic adenoma. It has malignant epithelial and stromal components with high rate of recurrence, metastatic spread and mortality (52). When this tumor metastasizes, both components almost always metastasize together. The carcinomatous component varies but may show adenocarcinoma, squamous cell carcinoma and undifferentiated carcinoma. In few cases specific salivary carcinoma phenotype like adenoid cystic carcinoma or salivary duct carcinoma are encountered. Sarcomatous elements are quite variable including chondrosarcoma, osteosarcoma, fibrosarcoma, malignant fibrous histiocytoma etc.

Carcinosarcoma is thought to develop de novo in the salivary gland. A study of loss of heterozygosity in tumor suppressor genes in cases of carcinosarcoma showed that mutational profiles for both types of malignant elements were similar. This supports the concept that all malignant elements of carcinosarcoma are derived from a common clonal precursor (51).

In a review of 5 series over a period of 40 years (53) only 18 cases (0.14%) of carcinosarcoma were reported out of a total of 12651 malignant tumors of salivary glands In cases of carcinoma sarcoma arising from minor salivary glands in aero-digestive tract the tumor should be differentiated from a spindle celled squamous cell carcinoma. The latter will show origin from the overlying squamous mucosa. The carcinosarcoma will show foci of adenocarcinoma and lack of origin from the mucosa. True malignant mixed tumor has a poor prognosis and 60% of the patients die of local recurrence and/or metastases within 2 to 3 years.

Carcinoma Ex-Pleomorphic Adenoma (CA-ex-PA)

(Carcinoma arising in Pleomorphic Adenoma)

This is a mixed tumor, in which second neoplasm develops from epithelial component and it fulfills criteria for malignancy. These include destruction of normal tissue, cellular anaplasia, atypical mitoses, abnormal organizational patterns like back to back gland arrangement and neoplastic cells in solid sheets. Benign mixed tumors may, on occasion, have focal areas of marked epithelial atypia. Therefore cellular atypia alone is insufficient for a definitive diagnosis of malignancy. When this tumor metastasizes, only the carcinoma component does so, benign component being not found in the metastatic deposit. 82% of Ca-ex-PA cases occur in major salivary glands and only 18% involve the minor salivary glands of upper aero-digestive tract.

Most frequent clinical presentation is a painless slowly growing mass and 15% have recent rapid growth with ulceration. In cases of CA-ex-PA tumor, the patients often have a long standing history of a salivary gland lesion which may have undergone multiple operations for recurrent pleomorphic adenoma. The tumor is usually poorly circumscribed and many are extensively infiltrative. Some tumors may be encapsulated and some well circumscribed. The proportion of benign and malignant components varies considerably and in some cases multiple sections will have to be studied to search for small remnants of typical pleomorphic adenoma. If there is a previous history of histologically proven benign mixed tumor present at the same site bearing malignancy, it can be classified as carcinoma arising in mixed tumor. The malignant component is most commonly a poorly differentiated adenocarcinoma, squamous cell carcinoma or even an undifferentiated carcinoma (Figure 42, 43). Salivary gland type carcinomas like adenoid cystic carcinoma, mucoepidermoid carcinoma, salivary duct carcinoma etc have also been reported as the malignant component of CA-ex-PA.

CA-ex-PA tumor should be classified as noninvasive (encapsulated}, minimally invasive (<_1.5 mm penetration in extra-capsular tissues) and invasive when infiltration is more than 1.5 mm. The first two subtypes have good prognosis. About 40-50% patients develop one or more recurrences even after wide local excision with contiguous lymph node dissection. The metastatic rate varies from series to series and up to 70% patients develop local or distant metastasis. The sites of distant metastases, in order of frequency, have been lung, spine, liver and brain.(54, 55).

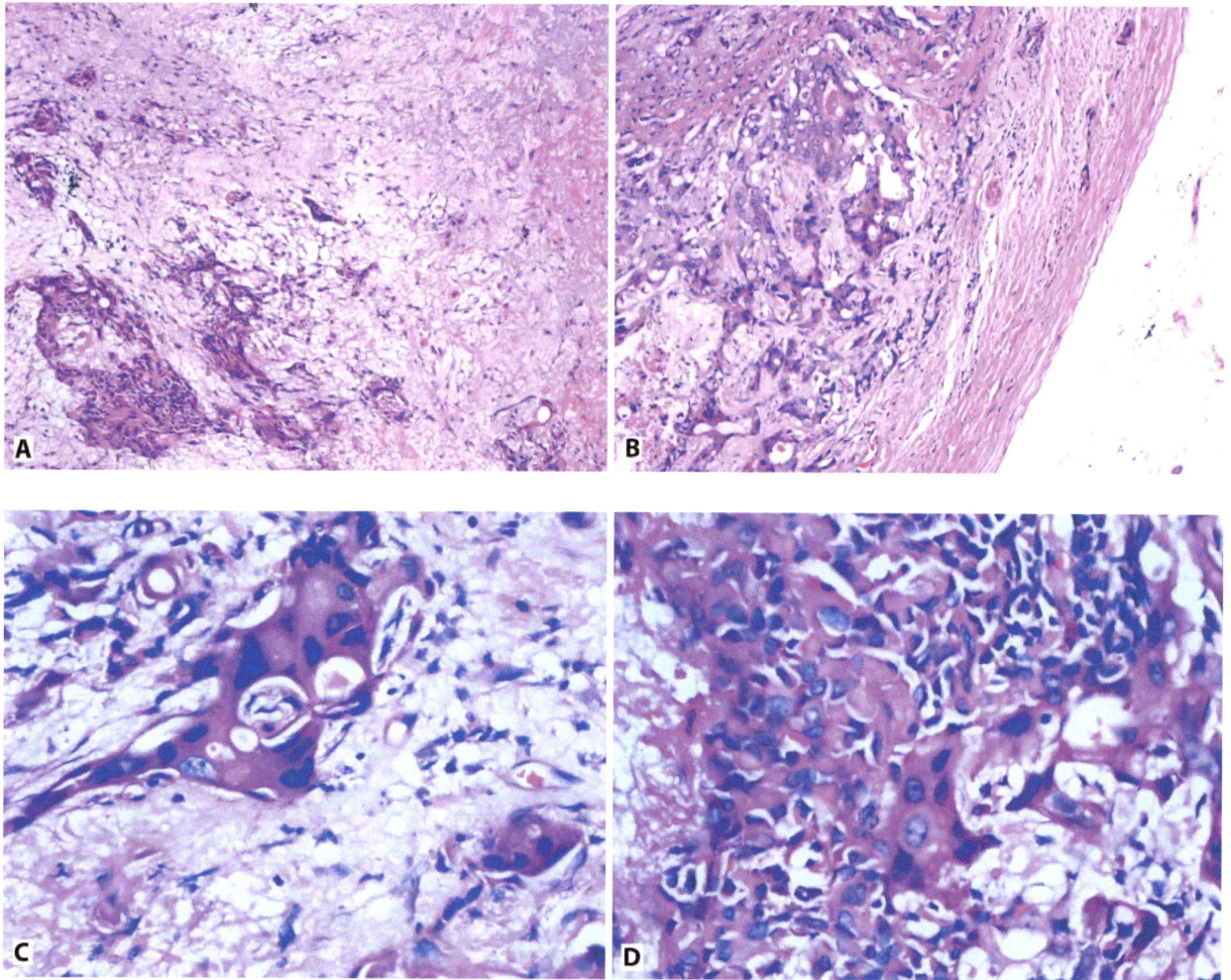

Figure 42 (A & B) myxomatous stromal background, (C & D) squamous cell carcinoma ex pleomorphic adenoma

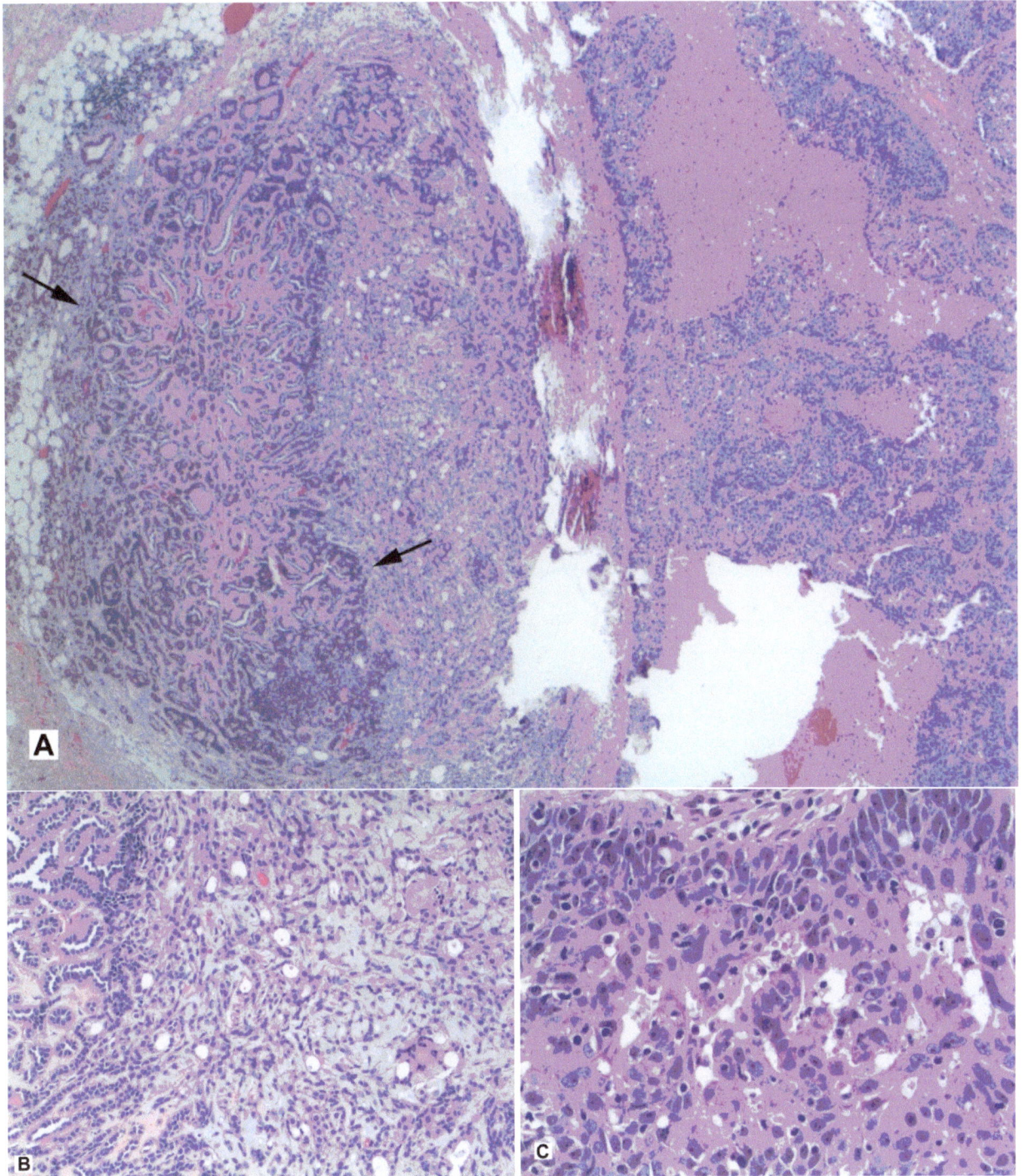

Figure 43 (A) Scanner view of carcinoma arising in the background of pleomorphic adenoma (arrows); (B) pleomorphic adenoma component; (C)showing high grade carcinomatous component

Metastasizing Benign Mixed Tumor (MZMT)

Metastasizing mixed tumor (MZMT) is a histologically benign pleomorphic adenoma that inexplicably manifests local or distant metastasis. Approximately only 40 cases have been reported as of 2000. It is akin to a metastasizing uterine leiomyoma or metastasizing giant cell tumor (osteoclastoma) of bone.

With a rare exception, all cases of MZMT have a history of two or more local recurrences of histologically benign pleomorphic adenoma. There are no morphological features that can reliably identify mixed tumors that will ultimately metastasize, although tumor longevity and tumor recurrence are clinical factors that strongly influence the likelihood of developing MZMT. Metastatic deposits have been identified in bone, lung, local lymph nodes, skin, kidney, brain etc and were discovered any where from 6 to 52 years (average 16 years) following the occurrence of the primary tumor. MZMTs have been associated with an overall mortality of 22% (56).

The subject of MMT has been most exhaustively studied by Gnepp (1993) and the incidence data for cumulated 60 recent series revealed 1352 carcinomas arising in mixed tumor out of a total of 24,527 mixed tumors, which comes to 5.5% prevalence of MZMT (53).

Neuroectodermal Neoplasms of Head & Neck

Under the rubric neuroectodermal tumors, there are two broad groups. Group 1 tumors are neuroendocrine carcinomas of various grades of malignancy and Group 2 tumors encompass those exhibiting neuronal differentiation. In 1993, the World Health Organization (WHO) divided laryngeal neuroendocrine neoplasms into carcinoid, atypical carcinoid and small cell carcinoma. There has been a consensus among the experts to replace the older terminology with a more realistic and easy to adapt nomenclature (see below).

Group 1: Neuroendocrine tumors	
Older Nomenclature	Current Nomenclature
Carcinoid	well differentiated neuroendocrine carcinoma
Atypical carcinoid	moderately differentiated neuroendocrine carcinoma
Small cell carcinoma	poorly differentiated neuroendocrine carcinoma ((a) small cell carcinoma (b) large cell carcinoma)

Neuroendocrine tumors are adequately described in the gastrointestinal system.

Group 2 neuroectodermal neoplasms, which display neural differentiation, are more varied and diverse. Some of these tumors will be discussed in this chapter.
Neuroectodermal Neoplasms
Olfactory neuroblastoma
Paraganglioma
PNET/Ewing's sarcoma
Malignant melanoma
Melanotic neuroectodermal tumor of infancy

Olfactory Neuroblastoma (ONB)

(Synonyms: Esthesioneuroblastoma, esthesioneurocytoma, esthesioneuroepithelioma, esthesioneuroma, olfactory placode tumor etc)

Definition and histogenesis

Esthesioneuroblastoma and olfactory neuroblastoma are two commonly used terms but currently the designation olfactory neuroblastoma is preferred. It is a rare, locally aggressive neuronal tumor thought to arise from olfactory membrane or olfactory placode (Placode: plate like thickening of embryonic ectoderm). The anatomical location extends from roof of nasal cavity to mid nasal septum and superior turbinate in fetus. Apart from this, histological, immunophenotypic and ultrastructural features suggest its origin in the neuronal or neuroendocrine cells of the olfactory epithelium. The latter is composed of bipolar sensory neurons, supporting cells and reserve (basal) cells. The reserve cells are mitotically active and presumed to be the progenitor of olfactory neuroblastoma (ONB). However, ONB differs from typical pediatric neuroblastoma of sympathetic nervous system, in that the characteristic N-myc amplification is not present. According to some studies, ONB belongs to the peripheral PNET family, since EWS/FLI1 fusion transcript was detected in this tumor. Yet another more detailed study failed to show EWS gene rearrangement in ONB in a series of 11 cases. CD 99 immunostain was also consistently negative. The histogenesis and nomenclature of olfactory neuroblastoma, thus, remains debatable (59, 59a, 60).

Presenting features of ONB include signs of nasal obstruction and epistaxis and occurrence in a broad age range with bimodal incidence peaks at about 15 and 55 years, unlike in the conventional childhood neuroblastoma. Cases of Cushing's syndrome arising from ectopic ACTH producing ONB have been reported. After successful surgical excision, the patient's symptoms are completely resolved and ACTH and cortisol levels greatly reduced (61, 62).

Histologically, the tumor exhibits well defined nesting pattern or sheet like growth pattern (Figure 44 A). In many areas the neoplastic cells are small and round with inconspicuous small nucleoli and minimal cytoplasm. Nuclear anaplasia is usually mild. The most helpful diagnostic feature is the presence of fibrillary background caused by interdigitating neuronal cell processes. In some cases, Homer-Wright rosettes (central fibrillary core and annular nuclear array) are encountered (Figure 44 B & C). The Flexner-Wintersteiner type rosettes, which are well formed acinar structures lined by tall columnar cells with basal nuclei and lumen delimitated by basal lamina (Figure 44 D) have been rarely described. The tumor cells express synaptophysin, NSE and chromogranin and in sharply demarcated nests, S100 positive cells are seen at the periphery. These cells show characteristic ultrastructural features of Schwann cells. A cases of predominant neuroblastic ONB (45 A-C) are described.

A small biopsy from a clinically suspected olfactory neuroblastoma may be difficult to interpret because of divergent differentiation in the form of focal glandular, squamous, melanocytic or myogenic cells observed in some cases of ONB. Immunohistochemistry will show positive staining for CK, EMA and HMB 45. Notwithstanding the putative neuronal histogenesis of ONB, its divergent differentiation puts the tumor well apart from neuroblastoma. There are reports of cases of ONB with adenocarcinoma, one case of ONB had a mixture of ganglioneuroblastoma and adenocarcinoma and another revealed neuroblastoma mixed with squamous cell carcinoma and small carcinoma. It is tempting to consider such cases to be malignant teratomas rather than ONB. However, none of the above reported cases had associated seminoma, choriocarcinoma or embryonal carcinoma component.

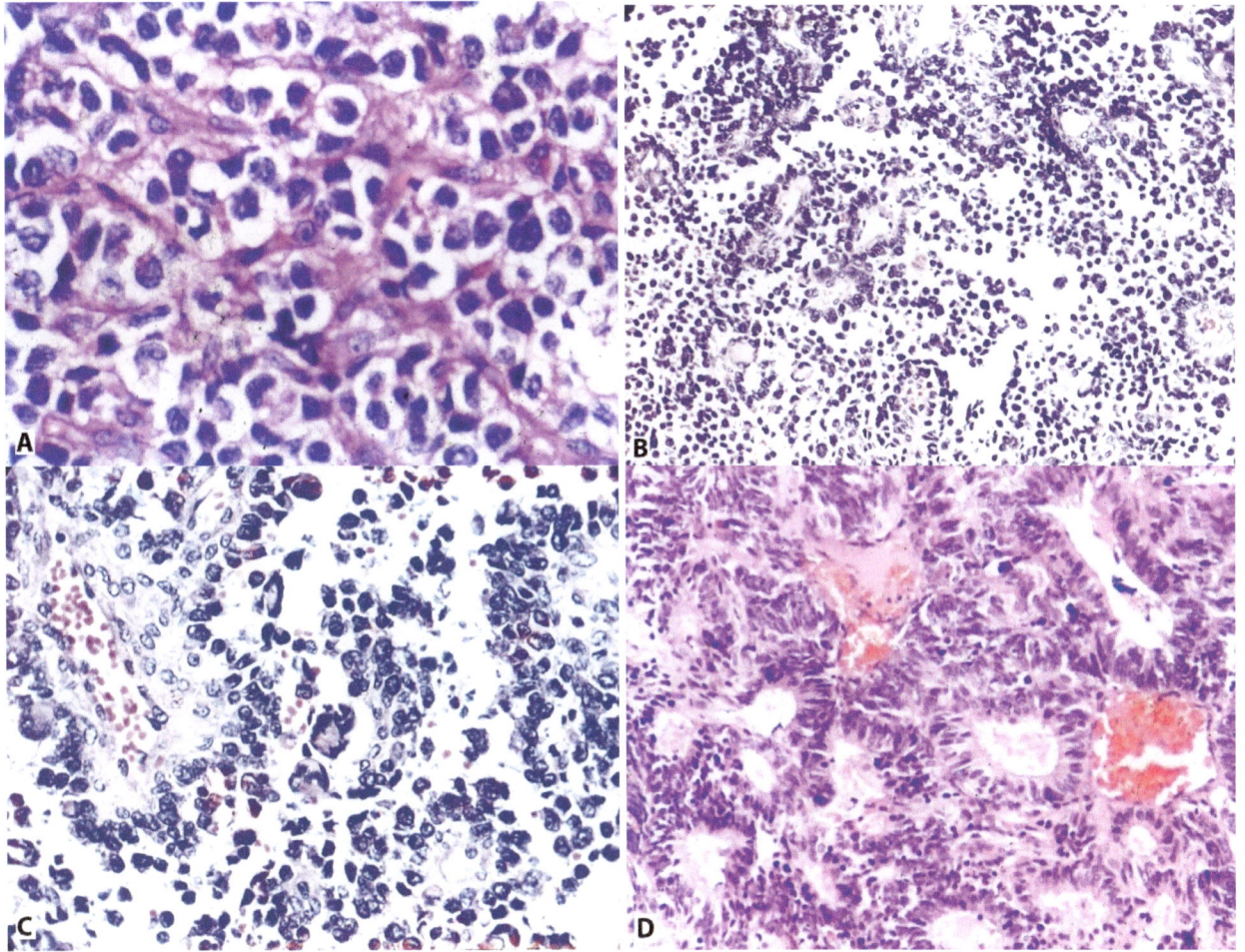

Figure 44 (A) large undifferentiated cells in sheets, (B & C) small undifferentiated cells forming rosettes and palisades around vascular stroma, (D) Flexner Wintersteiner rosettes

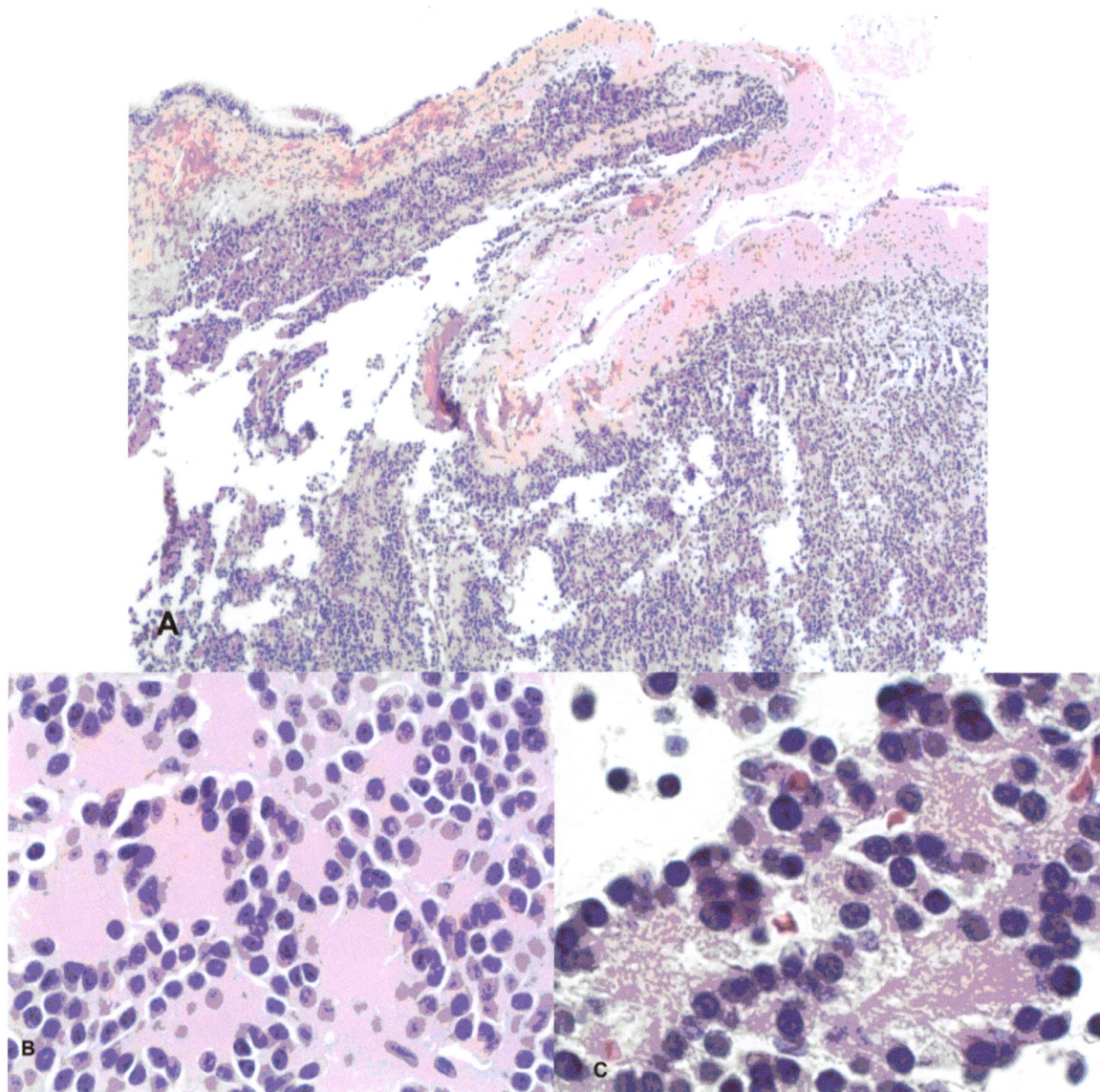

Figure 45 Olfactory neuroblastoma (A) scanner view of olfactory neuroblastoma covered with nasal respiratory epithelium; (B) rosette formation; (C) matrix of neuropil

Teratocarcinosarcoma

(Synonym: Malignant teratoma)

This rare tumor of sinonasal tract is characterized by a histologic combination of malignant teratoma and carcinosarcoma with triphasic growth pattern including epithelial, mesenchymal, and primitive neuroectodermal components (Figure 46 A-D). It is felt that teratocarcinosarcoma does not deserve status of a separate entity, since epithelial structures have also been frequently described in olfactory neuroblastoma in the literature (63).

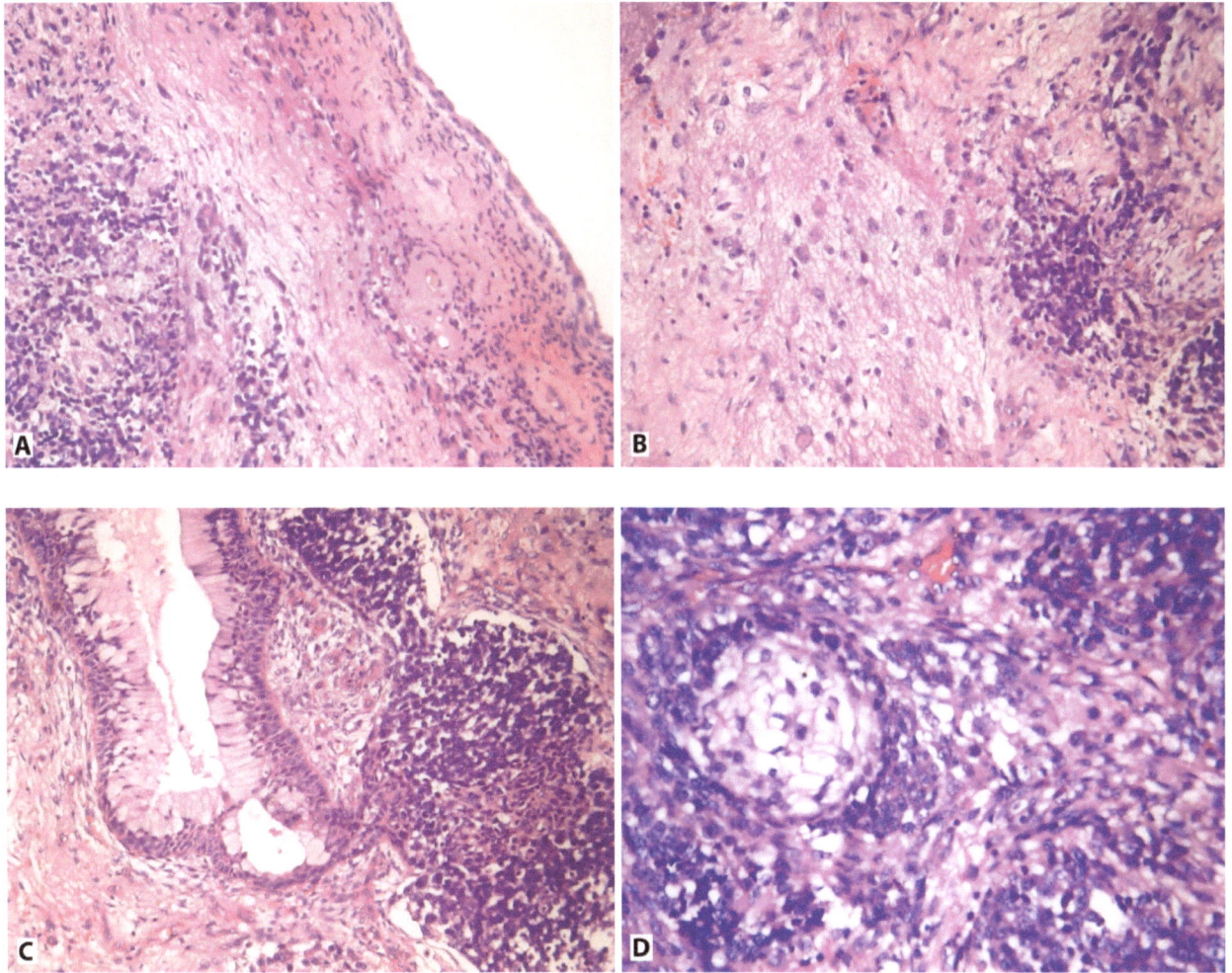

Figure 46 (A, B) predominant neuronal component with rich fibrillar network (C) unequivocal glandular differentiation and masses of undifferentiated apparent neuronal cells (D) an island of vacuolated squamous cells

Melanotic Neuroectodermal tumor of Infancy

(Synonyms: retinal analogue tumor, melanotic ameloblastotma, melanotic progonoma, congenital melanocarcinoma)

Melanotic neuroectodermal tumor of infancy is a rare tumor of neural crest origin that is commonly (70%) found in maxilla of infants and remaining elsewhere in head neck sites like mandible, skull, Dura mater or brain. These have also been reported in far flung sites, namely: epididymis, skin, uterus and mediastinum.

Morphologically it consists of a dual population of large and small cells forming alveolar or vague gland like structures embedded in a fibrotic stroma. The small cells resemble neuroblastoma cells and large cells often contain melanin pigment in the cytoplasm. Necrosis, pleomorphism and mitotic activity are rarely found. IHC reveals cytokeratin, HMB 45 and less commonly EMA in the large cells. Both large and small cells usually express NSE. In one reported case of pigmented maxillary lesion in a 3 month old infant elevated VMA level in urine was noted and it returned to normal after surgical excision of the lesion in toto. This clearly supports the neural origin of the tumor. The reproducible, characteristic, histological appearance of the lesion readily separates it from other small cell malignant tumors (57, 58).

Large majority of these tumors are cured if excised totally in the first instance. About 10% to 15% come back with local recurrence and roughly 5% develop metastases to regional nodes, liver or lungs.

Mucosal Malignant Melanoma of Head & Neck

Epidemiology

In a recent National Cancer Data Base report of 84,836 melanomas of all sites, head and neck mucosal melanomas comprised only 0.7%. The incidence of ocular melanoma is much higher than that of all mucosal melanomas. The reported incidence of mucosal melanoma across the world varies widely, being 0.2% to 10%, depending upon the ethnic and geographic differences. The proportion of mucosal melanoma is reportedly higher in Asians compared to that in Caucasians (64).

In our experience of 80 non-cutaneous malignant melanomas, 35 occurred in anorectal region, 29 in Head & Neck and 16 in lower female genital tract. Of the 29 cases in Head & Neck 9 occurred in eye ball, 8 in gums, 6 in nose, 2 in tonsils and 1 each in tongue and lip. In one large series of 115 cases of mucosal malignant melanoma 39 were present in anorectum, 30 in nasal cavity, 21 in genitourinary, 14 in oral cavity, 6 in upper gastrointestinal tract and 5 in maxillary sinus (65).

Unless the lesion is grossly pigmented one does not even think of occurrence of melanoma in mucosal sites. Some tumors have a little melanin pigment in few cells, which can be easily missed. The problem is further compounded by a broad spectrum of cytological appearance of melanoma; namely: epithelioid, spindle celled, rhabdoid, plasmacytoid, small celled etc.

In a series of 115 sinonasal melanomas, 38 (33%) were of amelanotic type (65). Thus, a constellation of diverse morphologic features and an absence of melanin pigment bring a large variety of head and neck neoplasms into the differential diagnosis. For a small round cell pattern the differential diagnosis includes olfactory neuroblastoma, PNET, Ewing's sarcoma, pituitary adenoma, non-Hodgkin's lymphoma, plasmacytoma, neuroendocrine carcinoma and mesenchymal chondrosarcoma. In case of pleomorphic appearance of the tumor, undifferentiated carcinoma, angiosarcoma, anaplastic large cell lymphoma and rhabdomyosarcoma should be considered .For spindle cell pattern the differential diagnosis includes malignant peripheral nerve sheath tumor, fibrosarcoma, malignant fibrous histiocytoma, leiomyosarcoma and synovial sarcoma. This exercise will entail application of a panel of antibodies, which include cytokeratin cocktail, Vimentin, S100, HMB 45, LCA, desmin, chromogranin, synaptophysin and CD 30.

Distinction of malignant melanoma from other less aggressive tumors is obviously of great therapeutic and prognostic importance. Once the possibility of melanoma is suspected its immunohistochemical identification is fairly easy. The presence of melanosomes in the tumor cells on electron microscopy is pathognomonic of melanoma. S-100 protein remains the most sensitive marker (positive in 95% of cases) for the diagnosis of melanoma, especially for desmoplastic and spindle cell type of melanoma. HMB 45 is a more specific but less sensitive (71% cases positive) marker than S-100 protein (Figure 47, 48).

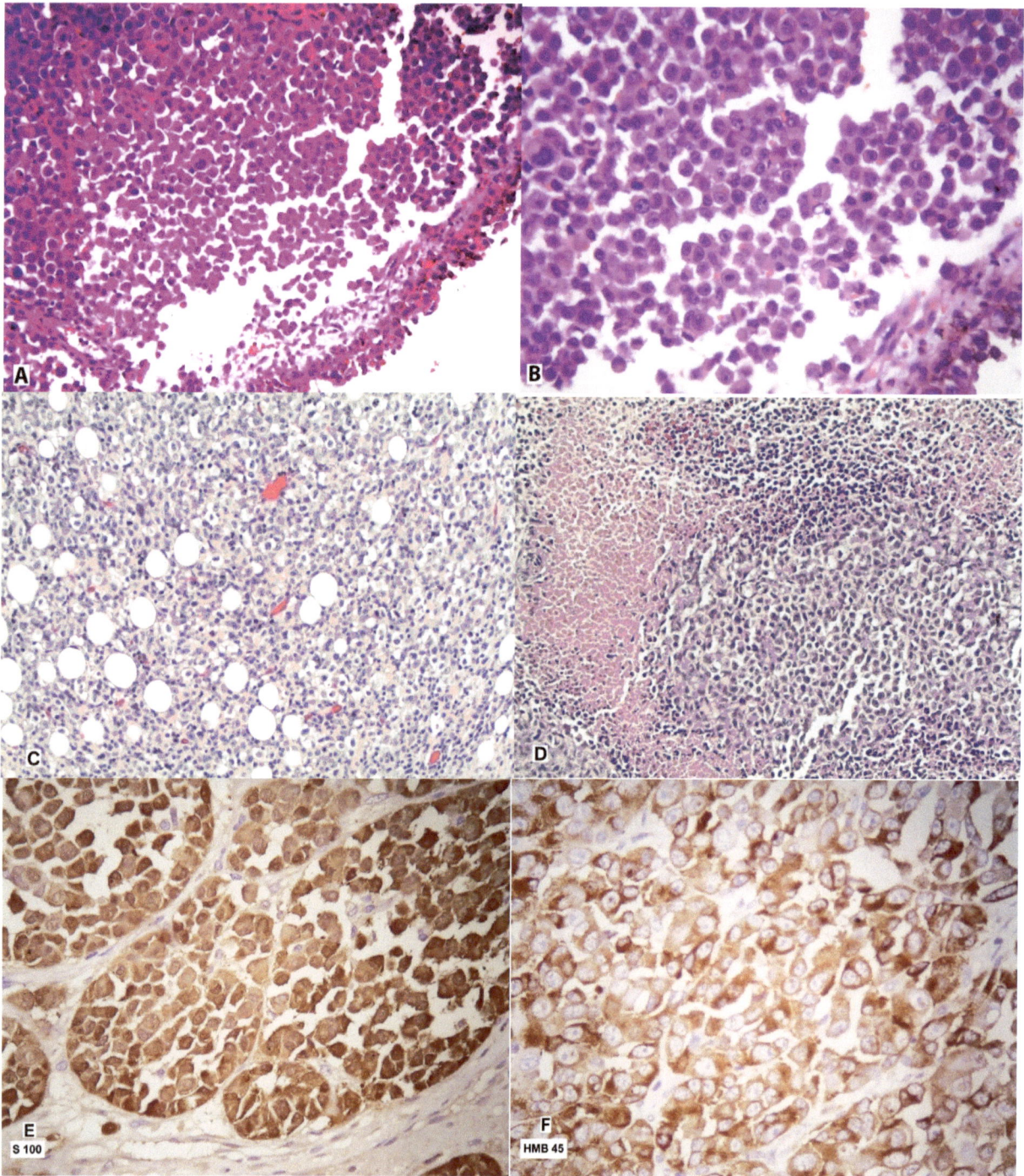

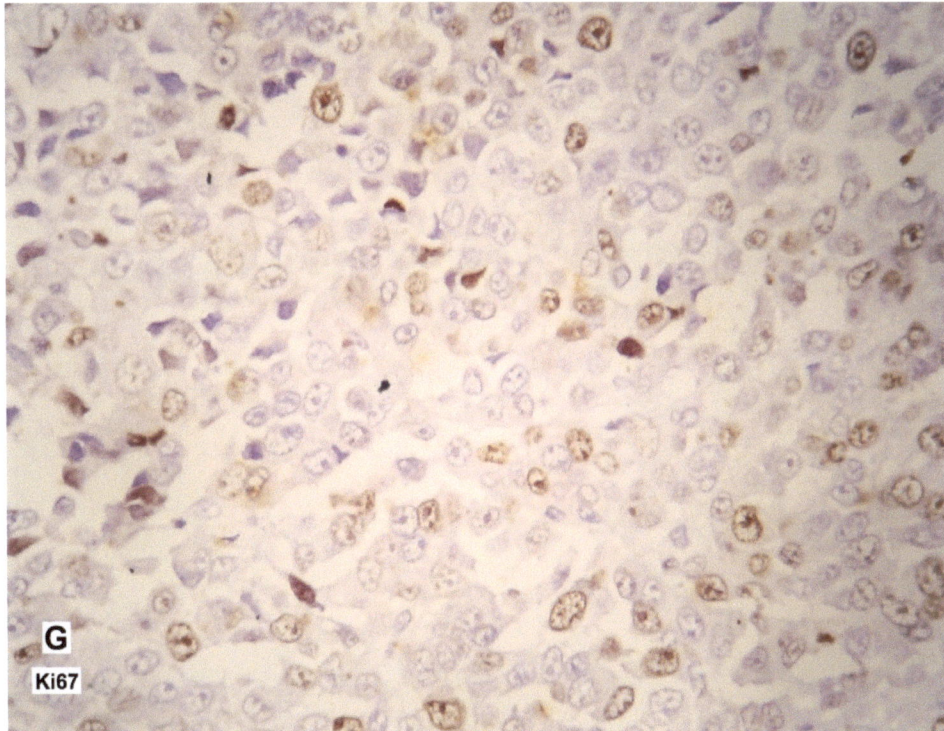

Figure 47 (A & B) amelanotic tumor with plasmacytoid features, note overlying respiratory epithelium of nasal cavity; (C) amelanotic cells infiltrating fatty tissue; (D)patchy tumor necrosis (E & F) strong staining for S 100 and HMB 45 melanoma markers respectively; (G) ki 67 decorates many tumor cell nuclei(high proliferation index)

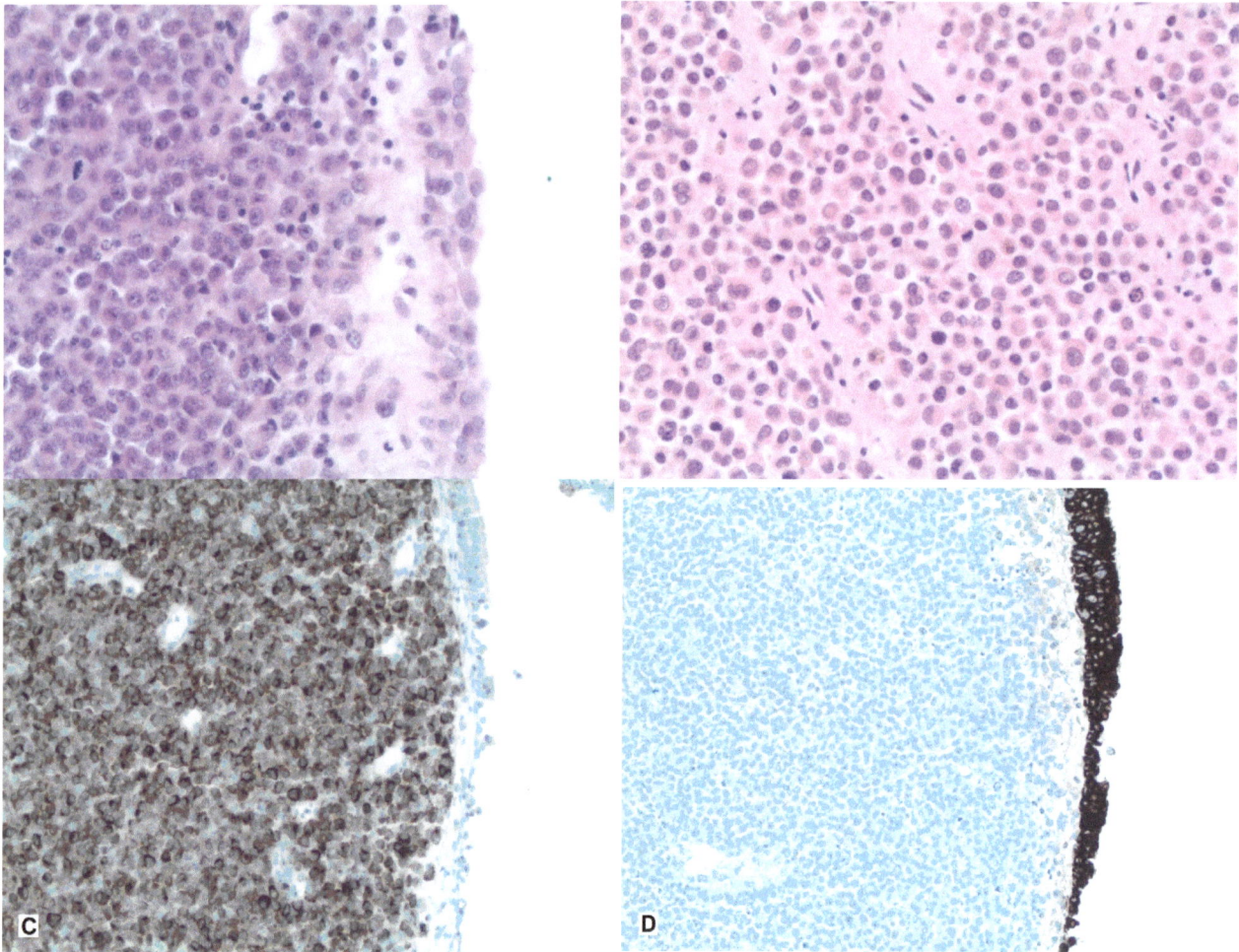

Figure 48 (A) another case of amelanotic melanoma with respiratory mucosa; (B) plasmacytoid appearance; (C) strong staining for HMB-45; (D), tumor negative for cytokeratin- note positive overlying nasal mucosa

There are other specific markers like Melan A and particularly T311 (tyrosinase), which approaches the sensitivity of anti S-100 protein. T311 was found to be the most useful marker in the diagnosis of mucosal melanomas of the head and neck region. The presence of tyrosinase antigen in all sinonasal and nearly all oral mucosal melanomas suggests that it may be an attractive target for immunotherapeutic treatment against mucosal melanoma (66).

Currently, surgery (wide local resection) is the treatment of choice and radiation/ chemotherapy have little, if any role, to play. Mucosal malignant melanomas are aggressive tumors with a disease free 5 year survival of 31.3% as compared to 5 year survival rate of 88% for cutaneous malignant melanoma. The 10 year survival for mucosal melanoma is reported to be 22.6%. Vascular invasion, necrosis and polymorphous tumor cell population are three histological parameters that have statistically significant predictive value and imply a less favorable prognosis (67).

Pathology of Parasympathetic Paraganglia

Paraganglia are dispersed neuroendocrine organs, occurring as anatomically discrete bodies, composed of catecholamine secreting cells derived from the neural crest. Paraganglia are of two types: Sympathetic (sympathetico-adrenal system) and parasympathetic (located along the distribution of glassopharyngeal and vagus nerves). They have been given a variety of names and there is some confusion about the nomenclature because of significant overlap. WHO classification defines pheochromocytoma as a tumor of chromaffin cells of the 'adrenal medulla' and all others are extra-adrenal paragangliomas. This restriction of pheochromocytoma to the adrenal medulla is a bit arbitrary because few parasympathetic paragangliomas also secrete epinephrine or non-epinephrine and can legitimately be labeled as pheochromocytoma. However, this occurrence is rare or anecdotal and most parasympathetic paragangliomas are not secretary. Following schematic view of defined parasympathetic paraganglia should be helpful.

Anatomical sites of parasympathetic paraganglia include jugulotympanic, vagal, carotid body, larynx and aortopulmonary as shown below.

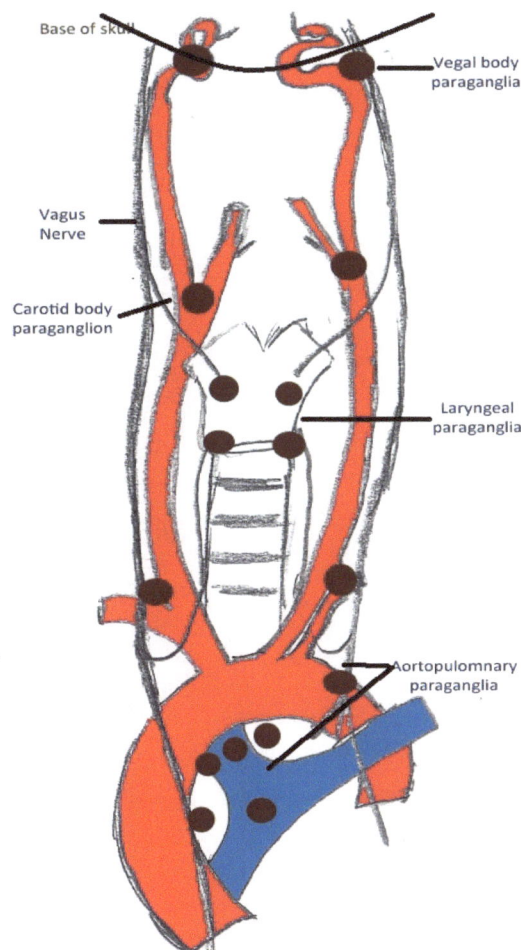

Anatomic distribution of parasympathetic paraganglia

Autonomus nervous system

Paraganglia

PARASYMPATHETIC
Jugulo-tympanic
Vagal
Carotid
Laryngeal
Aortico-pulmonary
Urinary Bladder

Glossary of Terms

Glomus: "a ball" in Latin; the term applied to various paraganglia of head and neck: glomus caroticum, glomus jugulare, glomus tympanicum glomus intravagale etc Use of this term glomus for paraganglia should be avoided.

Glomus: The term is also used for specialized arterio-venous anastomoses located in nailbed and elsewhere in skin involved in local thermal regulation.

Chromaffin Reaction: (1) Paraganglioma tissue exposed to fixatives containing dichromate salts or potassium iodate turn brown, a reaction seen grossly and also microscopically.

(2) Paraganglioma tissue section in fresh frozen state exposed to formaldehyde will emit fluorescence, if catecholamines are present in cells.

Chromaffin Paraganglioma: Catecholamine secreting tumor, pheochromocytoma and very rarely parasympathetic paraganglioma.

Non-Chromaffin Paraganglioma: Almost all cases of head and neck paraganglioma will show negative staining for catecholamines (no brown color).

Chemodectoma: The term used for tumors of chemoreceptor paraganglia, namely; carotid body and aortico-pulmonary body. These are baroreceptors, which are important in ventilatory compensation in chronic respiratory diseases with impaired pulmonary gas exchange

Features common to paragangliomas

1) Medium to large cuboidal cells in cohesive 'zellballen' arrangement.
2) Rich sinusoidal vascular supporting network giving an organoid pattern
3) NSE, Synaptophysin and Chromogranin A positive in cytoplasm of chief cells
4) S-100 positive for sustentacular spindle cells at the edge of cell balls (Figure 52c).
5) Electron microscopy: neurosecretory granules with uniform central round electron dense core and a narrow halo (70-200 nm in size), a hallmark of chief cells
6) A small biopsy may be difficult to interpret and the differential diagnosis depends upon the anatomical site of the tumor.

7) Presence of nuclear pleomorphism and even mitosis not diagnostic of malignancy.

8) Metastasis to lymph nodes or distant sites is the only reliable criteria for malignancy

Table 14: Parasympathetic Paragangliomas (n=120) Author's series (1970-2005)	
Jugulo-tympanic	45
Vagal	2
Carotid body tumor	20
Aortico pulmonary	3
Retroperitoneal*	39
Urinary bladder*	9
Prostate*	1
Paraduodenal*	1

Jugulo-Tympanic (JTP) Paraganglia:

Paraganglia have been demonstrated in adventitia of jugular bulb, tympanic branch of glossopharyngeal nerve and auricular branch of vagus nerve. In a review of 316 Jugulo-tympanic paragangliomas female: male ratio was 66:19 and average age at diagnosis 49 years. In another series of 231 cases the female: male ratio was 6:1 with an average age of 55 years. Jugular paraganglioma involves the temporal bone at the base of the skull and may grow within petrous bone with intracranial extension in the middle cranial fossa, at times. Large tympanic paragangliomas can fill the middle ear cavity, engulf osseous chain and bulge to form a middle ear polyp. Few cases of functionally active JTP have been reported. Histologically, these tumors tend to be highly vascular with prominent vessels and sinusoids. The differential diagnosis includes hemangioma, hemangiopericytoma and even meningioma for a JTP protruding in the cranial cavity. The chief cells of JTP are often small and even spindly and form inconspicuous nests. JTP is locally aggressive neoplasm but metastasis is quite rare and was found to be as low as 1.9% (68). Johnston and others reported a case of recurrent JTP, which developed regional metastases 10 years after initial diagnosis and metastasized to spine 3 years later. The review found only 20 documented cases of metastases of JTP (69).

Vagal Paraganglioma:

Vagal body paraganglia are multiple dispersed collections of paraganglial cell nests located at or just inferior to ganglion nodosum of the vagus nerve. The tumor may form a fusiform mass along the nerve or a global shape with attachment at the base of the skull. A variety of cranial palsies can be present, the most common being paresis of the vagus nerve leading to vocal cord dysfunction, horseness or dysphagia, and rarely ipsilateral Horner's syndrome. Many cases of catecholamine releasing vagal paragangliomas have been reported with signs and symptoms of pheochromocytoma (70, 71). A few VPs with dumbbell shaped extension through jugular foramen have been described. These had to be treated by suboccipital craniotomy for total excision. In one series of 36 tumors of cervical vagus nerve 18 (50%) were VPs and others nerve sheath tumors (72). Henrich et al (73) reviewed 141 cases from the literature and found 15 malignant ones with metastases in cervical nodes and 4 cases had metastases to lungs and bones..

Carotid Body Paraganglioma (CBP)

The carotid body paraganglia, located at the bifurcation of the common carotid artery, is a structure about the size of a grain of wheat. It has a regulatory function in conditions of hypoxia. Persons living in high altitude develop hyperplasia of carotid body paraganglia and paragangliomas in head and neck occur 10 times more frequently than in persons living at sea level. Patients suffering from chronic hypoxia as in chronic obstructive pulmonary disease and congenital heart disease also show high incidence of paraganglioma. (74, 75, 76, 77))

Carotid body paraganglioma is rare but occurs as a rather common member of head and neck paraganglioma family. CBP is usually encountered in adults in the fifth decade of life with a slight preponderance of female patients. In a multicentric review of 95 cases (78), majority (98%) presented with a mass in neck and often pressure symptoms of cranial nerve deficits. Nearly 18% of cases were bilateral and 4.2% were malignant. These tumors are usually well demarcated with a fibrous pseudocapsule, an average size of 3.8 cm (1.8 to 8.5 cm) and made up of light tan meaty tissue (Figure 49 A) The histological features are quite diagnostic and include typical "Zell balen pattern and sustentacular cells strongly expressing S 100 staining (Figure 49 B & C). Gruferman and others reported a case of CBP in two sisters and presented a literature review on epidemiological information on 88 familial and 835 non-familial (sporadic) cases (79, 80, 81).

Table 15 : Familial and non-familial carotid body tumors (data from Reference 80-Gruferman et al		
	Familial	Non-familial
F:M ratio	1.0	0.7
Av. Age	40.6	42.5
Bilaterality	31.8% (28/88)	4.2% (37/835)
Malig. Bilateral	3.6% (1/28)	0% (0/37)
Malig. Unilateral	2.0% (1/51)	12.6% (90/718)

Malignancy in CBP is based on the following: adherence to surrounding structures and incorporation of nerves, encirclement of carotid vessels, growth up to base of skull, capsular invasion and invasion of the arterial wall, including the media. Morphological criteria correlating with malignant behavior are not well defined. In one study a combination of mitotic activity, necrosis and vascular invasion were analyzed but the findings were inconclusive (80). However, now it is universally accepted that presence of metastasis is the only admissible criteria in the diagnosis of malignancy in CBP or any type of paraganglioma. Metastatic tumors most often involve regional nodes, bones, lungs and rarely other site like liver, pancreas, skin, brain etc.(82, 82, 83)

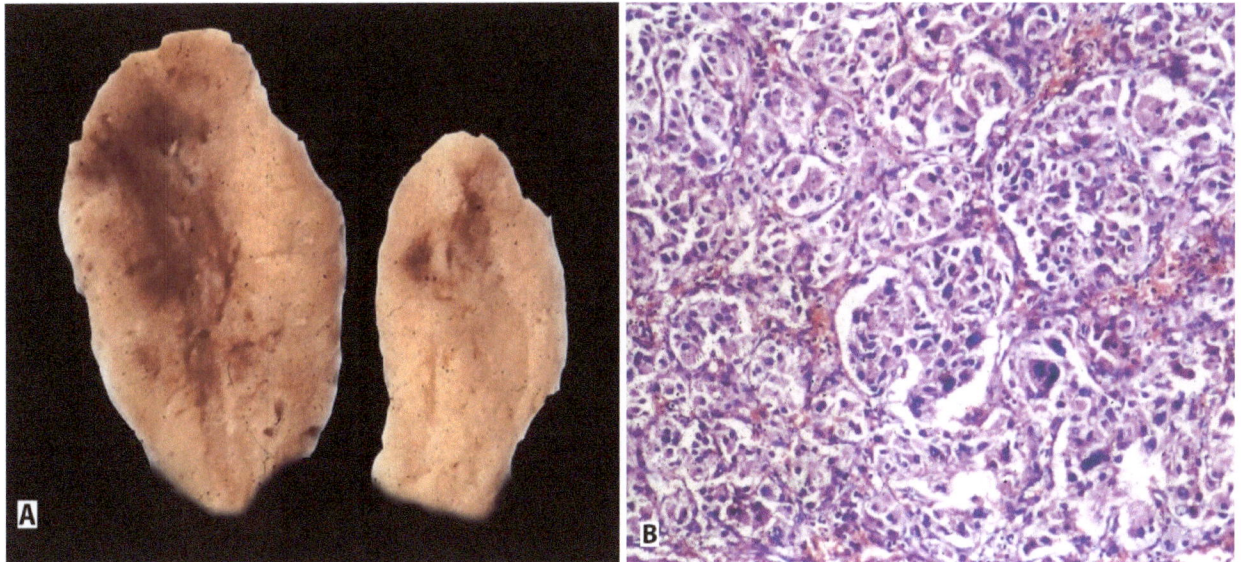

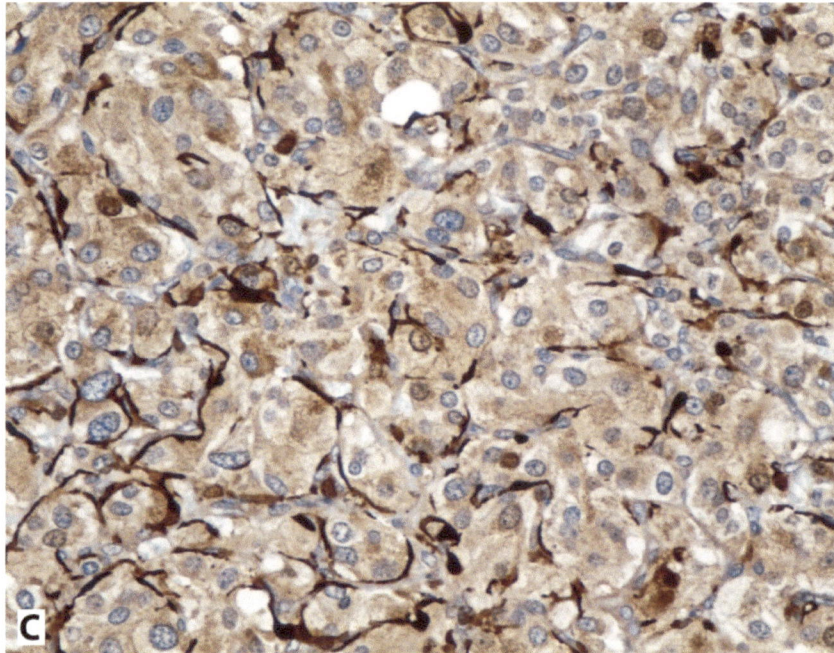

Figure. 4 (A) Carotid body tumor (B) typical "zellballen" pattern of cells of a paraganglioma (C) Scattered sustentacular cells positive with S 100 immunostaining

Laryngeal Paraganglioma

Paragangliomas arise from paraganglia occurring in false vocal cord and subglottic larynx and present as very vascular (red) submucosal tumors. The one in supraglottic region gives rise to hoarseness and dysphagia and the subglottic one can cause obstruction to the airway. Laryngeal paraganglioma is a rare tumor and about 76 cases have been reported to date. A striking female predominance (3:1) is noted (84). The most formidable problem is to histologically distinguish laryngeal paraganglioma from typical carcinoid, atypical carcinoid and medullary thyroid carcinoma. In fact all alleged malignant paraganglioma at this site are probably atypical carcinoid tumors, which have been misdiagnosed. Therefore accurate diagnosis is of great therapeutic significance. The paragangliomas respond well to surgical excision and the prognosis is far better than that of atypical carcinoid tumors. Radical neck dissection for lymph nodes is necessary for the treatment of the latter. The distinction between the two is effectively achieved by immunohistochemical tests. (85)

Aortico-Pulmonary Paraganglioma (APP)

There are small collections of paraganglia located at the various sites, both dorsal and ventral, at the base of the heart in relation to the great vessels. Aortico-Pulmonary paragangliomas (Figure 50 arising from these areas can cause hoarseness, dysphagia, chest pain and rarely hemoptysis and even superior vena cava syndrome. There is slight preponderance of female patients and the average tumor size is about 7.5 cm. APP has been reported to have involved pericardium or the heart directly (86, 87, 88). The frequency of metastasis has been estimated to be 13% to 20% (89). However, greater problem is the high incidence of unresectability due to direct involvement of vital structure in the mediastinum. In one review of mediastinal paragangliomas, 16 of 35 cases had important morbidity or death (89)

Pulmonary paraganglioma (88, 90) is indeed rare and there are a few cases reports. According to Lack (88) convincing illustrations are often lacking and it is difficult to differentiate paraganglioma from a far more common broncho-pulmonary carcinoid.

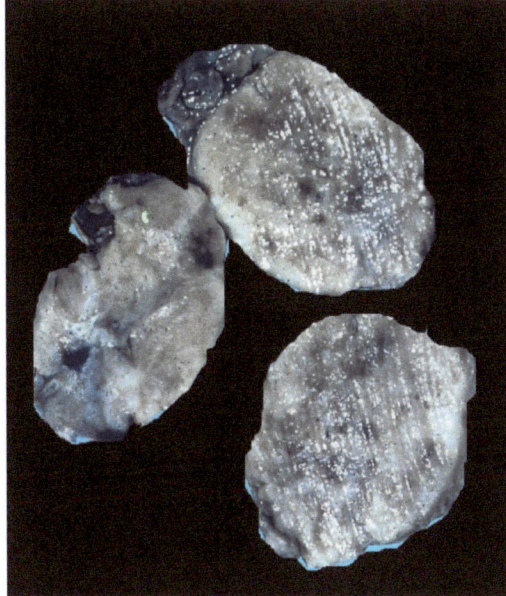

(Figure.50) Aortico-pulmonary paraganglioma

The subject of extradrenal sympathetic paragangliomas is described in the chapter on endocrine tumors.

Mesenchymal (Soft Tissues and Bones) Tumors of Head & Neck

Soft tissue tumors are virtually ubiquitous but relatively uncommon in head and neck region, accounting for only 5%-10% of all soft tissue tumors in the body. Each and every histological type of soft tissue tumors, both benign and malignant, can occur in this region. Hemangioma and nerve sheath tumor are often seen and rarely even a lipoma is encountered (Figure 53). It should be borne in mind that a spindle cell amelanotic melanoma and sarcomatous spindle cell squamous carcinoma are more frequently seen than mesenchymal spindle cell sarcoma. Immunohistochemistry should be performed for a definitive diagnosis. Any space occupying lesion (neoplastic or otherwise, benign or malignant) can raise serious clinical or radiological concern for malignancy. This is because of compression or erosion of adjacent structures leading to dramatic symptomatology like proptosis of the eye or distortion of facial features.

Most publications of malignant soft tissue tumors involving head and neck sites are single case reports. In adults, some soft tissue tumors occur in the following site specific groups:

-Neck (including pharynx and larynx): liposarcoma, MPNST & synovial sarcoma

-Skin of face and scalp: angiosarcoma and dermatofibrosarcoma

-Sinonasal tract: Nerve sheath tumors, hemangiopericytoma and solitary fibrous tumor

-Oral cavity: Rhabdomyosarcoma (particularly common in children and adults), leiomyosarcoma

A vast majority of soft tissue tumors arising in head and neck are not truly distinctive to this region, with the notable exception of nasopharyngeal angiofibroma and sinonasal hemangiopericytoma (91). A few soft tissue tumors encountered in our practice are also illustrated here.

Lipoma of Tongue

Lipoma of tongue is rare but there is no diagnostic difficulty. The case is illustrated to show that soft tissue tumors are ubiquitous and most are not specific for an anatomical site.

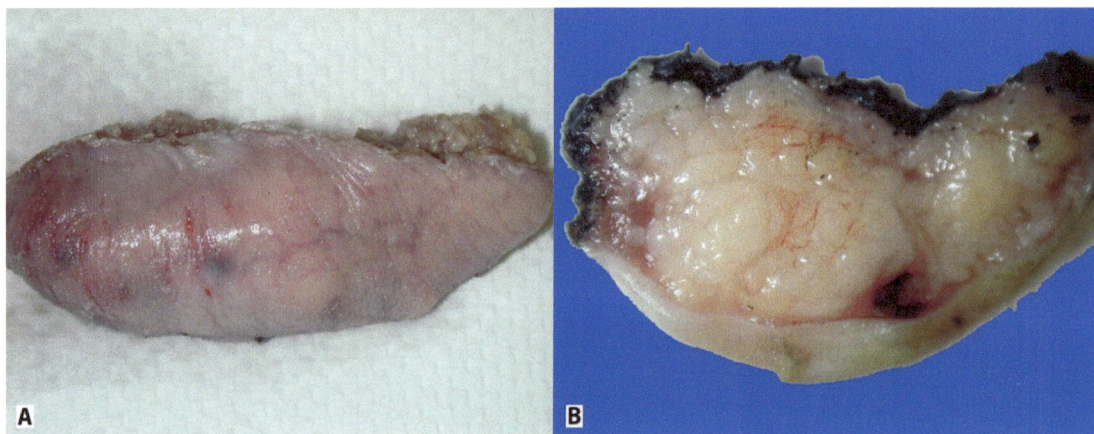

Figure 53 Lipoma of tongue: (A) mucosal surface, (B) undersurface showing lobules of adipose tissue

Nasopharyngeal Angiofibroma:

This lesion accounts for 0.5% of head and neck tumors, occurs almost exclusively in males at an age of about 15 years exhibiting intracranial extension in 10% to 20% cases and recurrence rate as high as 50% (92,93) (Figure   A-C). The tumor is located in posterior-lateral nasal wall near the sphenoid-palatine foramen, nasopharynx or pterygopalatine fossa. It can extend to middle cranial fossa along pterygoid process, erode sphenoid sinus and involve pituitary. Recurrent epistaxis and nasal obstruction are the most common symptoms.

The tumor is composed of an intricate mixture of vessels and fibrous stroma. This varies from loose and edematous with stellate fibroblasts and mast cells to a dense acellular highly collagenized tissue. The vessels vary from capillary size to venous size; the venous channels are usually dilated or

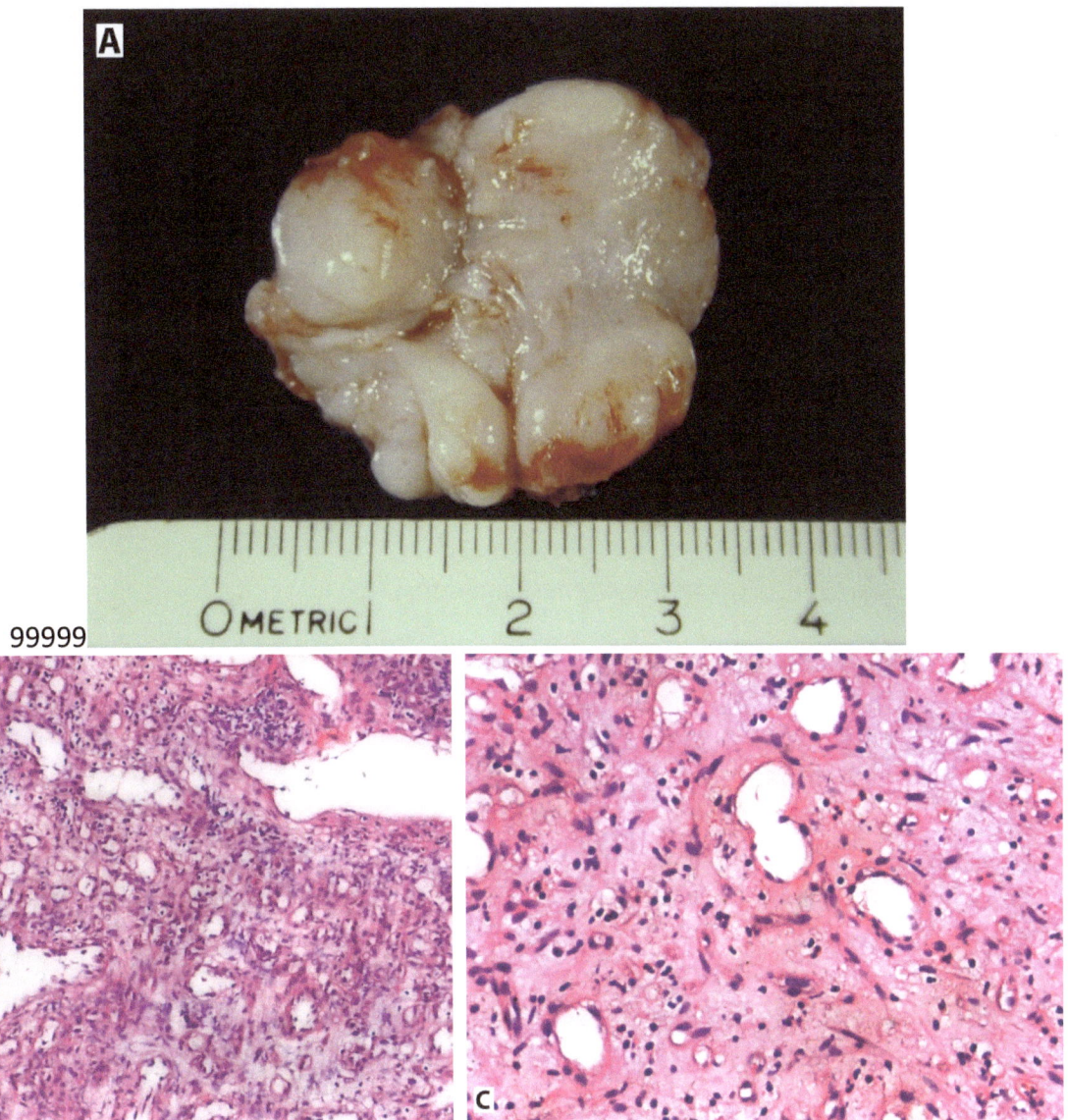

Figure 54 (A) well circumscribed soft to firm whitish lobulated 3 cm polypoid mass (B,C) tumor consists of numerous ectatic thin walled vascular channels separated by edematous stroma of short spindle cells tumor

tortuous and have irregular or deficient smooth muscle (Figure 54) It is important to distinguish angiofibroma from capillary hemangioma because of a different natural history of these lesions. Despite the frequent recurrence and local destruction of the surrounding tissues, the nuclear features are benign, except nuclear pleomorphism without mitosis in few cases. Immunocytochemical studies with antibodies to androgen (AR), estrogen (ER) and progesterone (PR) were carried out on 24 cases of angiofibroma. Positive stromal and endothelial nuclear immunostaining for AR was found in 18 out of 24 cases (75%) and for PR in only 2 of 24 (8%) cases. None of the cases was positive for estrogen (ER). These results provide a direct evidence for the presence of androgens in angiofibroma, which might help to explain the unique clinico-pathologic features of these tumors (94).

Hemangiopericytoma:

Vascular neoplasms, particularly hemangiomas, are quite common in sino-nasal tract. The less common hemangiopericytoma is of interest because of its biological behavior, difficult diagnostic problem in few cases and debatable histogenesis. Histologically, sheets of evenly spaced oval and fusiform cells, often in parallel, are arranged around blood vessels (Figure 55 A, B). These are thin walled and vary in size from large clefts or tightly compressed spaces with inconspicuous lining endothelial cells, discernible only after immunostains for endothelial cells. Nuclei tended to be uniform and cytological banal, with one or more small nucleoli. Immunohistochemistry is not a specific diagnostic feature, as only vimentin is almost always positive. Ultra structurally the presence of basal lamina around individual perivascular stromal cells and separating theses from the vessel wall was a consistent and virtually diagnostic finding. A review of literature showed that high local recurrence rates, late recurrences and low rates of metastasis were features characteristic of this tumor. Nuclear anaplasia is rarely encountered and this cannot account for the biological behavior. However, in one series of 106 cases of hemangiopericytoma of soft tissues the predictive factors for unfavorable outcome included nuclear atypia, necrosis, 4 or more mitoses per 10 HPF and size greater or equal to 6.5 cm (95). The tumor is discussed in detail in Chapter 4 on soft tissue tumors.

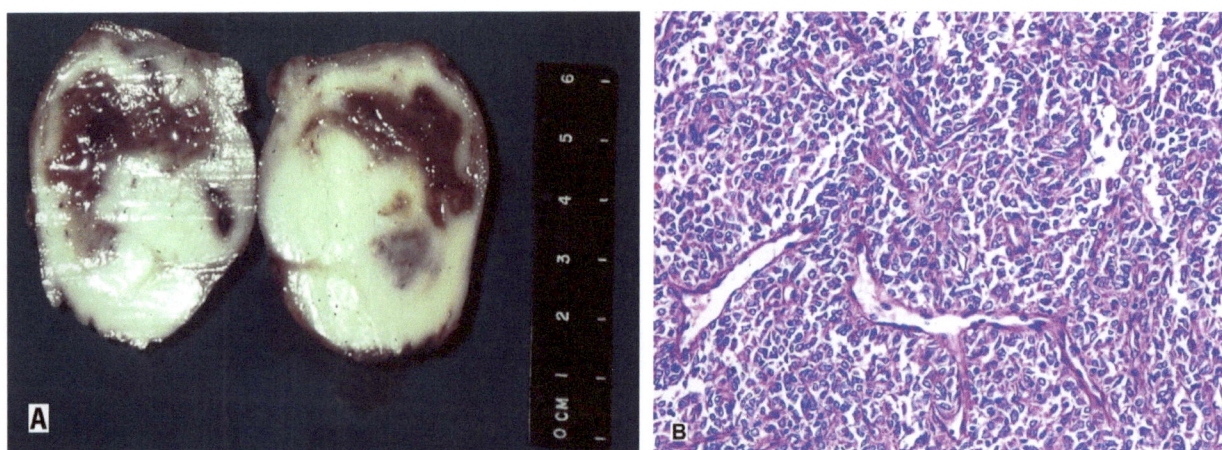

Figure 55 (A) Circumscribed oval whitish mass in nose with reddish discoloration. (B) plump oval and spindle shaped pericytes are arranged around thin walled vascular channels

Peripheral Nerve Sheath Tumor

These tumors are not uncommonly seen in sinonasal tract. The Schwannomas at this site are not encapsulated unlike all those ubiquitously occurring in the soft tissues of musculo--skeletal system. The malignant peripheral nerve sheath tumors (MPNST) are the most common primary spindle cell sarcomas in head and neck. It occurs mainly in adults and has a predilection for the sinonasal tract (Figure 56 A-D).

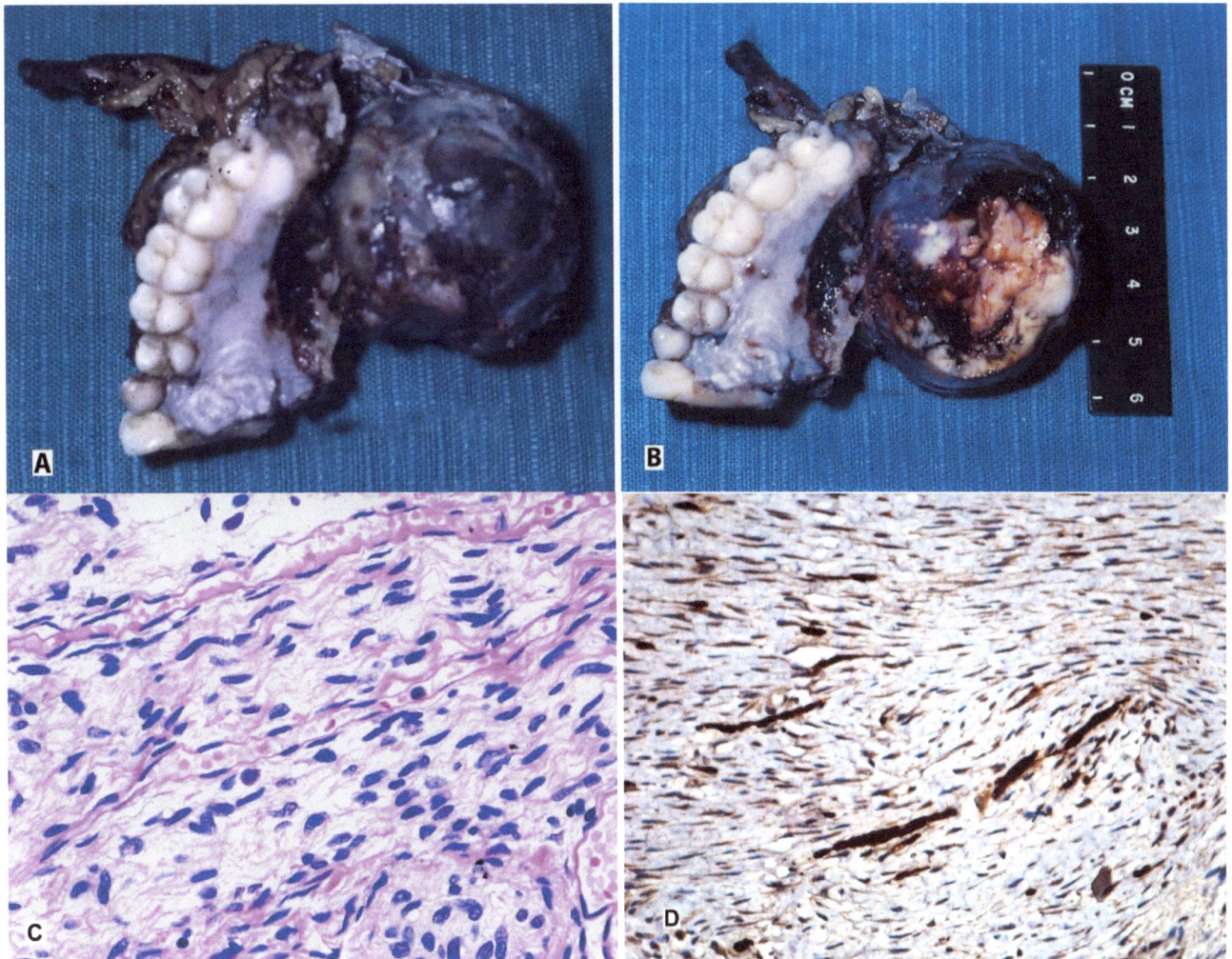

(Figure 56) (A & B) well encapsulated alignant peripheral nerve sheath tumor (MPNST) involving right maxilla; (C) loose sheets of spindly cells bearing wavy nuclei; (D) S 100 is strongly positive in nuclei

Rhabdomyosarcoma

This is the most common round cell malignant tumor occurring in children and adolescents and may be located in orbit, nasopharynx, sinonasal tract, oral cavity, middle ear and neck. Histologically, this tumor presents features of alveolar or embryonal type of rhabdomyosrcoma. Its differentiation from other malignant round cells is difficult without the aid of immunohistochemistry or electron microscopy (Figure 57 A-D).

embryonal – alternating hypercellular and hypocellular fields with myxoid or sparsely collagenized stroma; tumor cells have scanty cytoplasm, small, round/oval nuclei; may have occasional larger cells with abundant, deeply eosinophilic cytoplasm and cross striations

alveolar – fibrous septa lined by single row of tumor cells with additional tumor cells between the septa; may have multinucleated tumor cells, solid areas at periphery and clear cell change due to glycogen (PAS+)

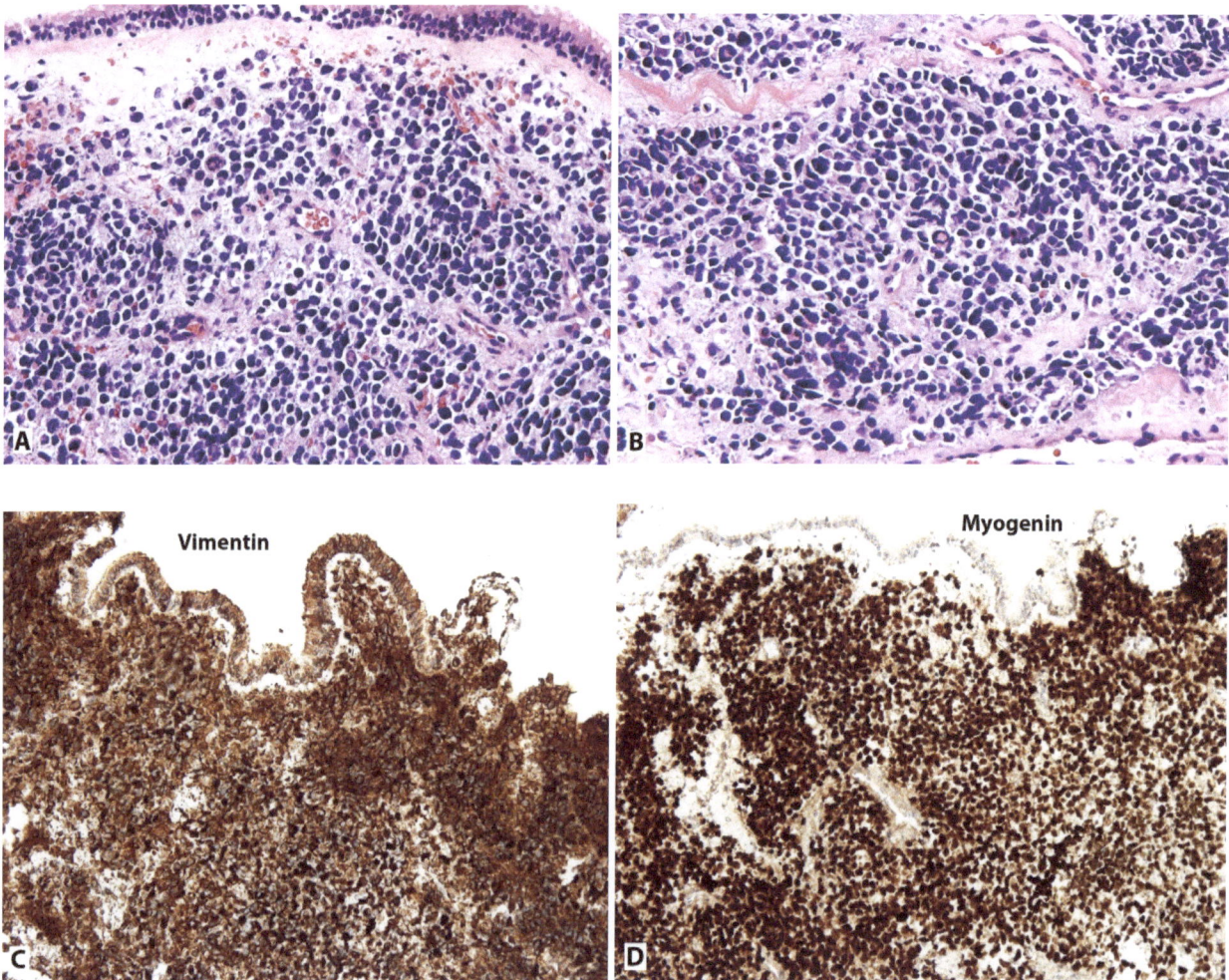

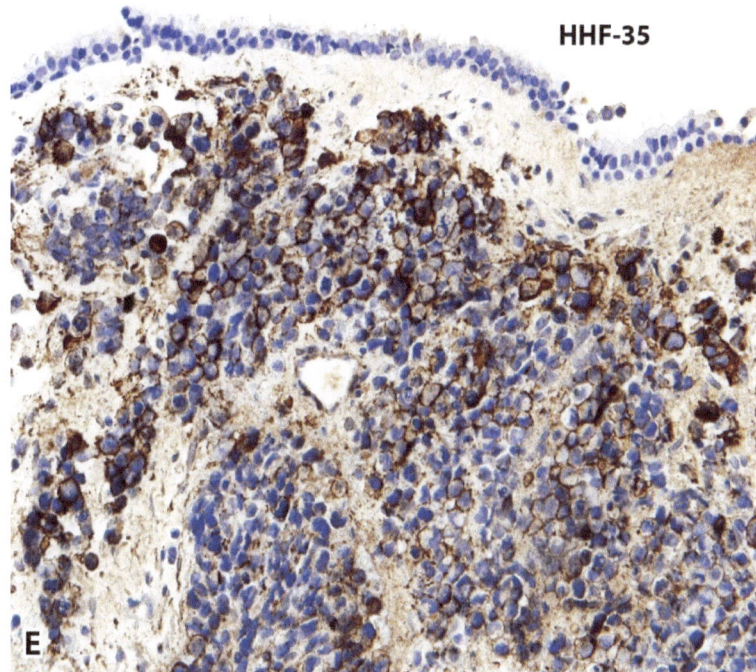

Figure 57 (A & B) Embryonal rhabdomyosarcoma of sinonasal tract in an 11 year old female: note loose sheets of undifferentiated small cell tumor with overlying nasal mucosa, (C) vimentin strongly expressed, (D & E) markers(myogenin and HHF-35) for skeletal muscle differentiation are positive

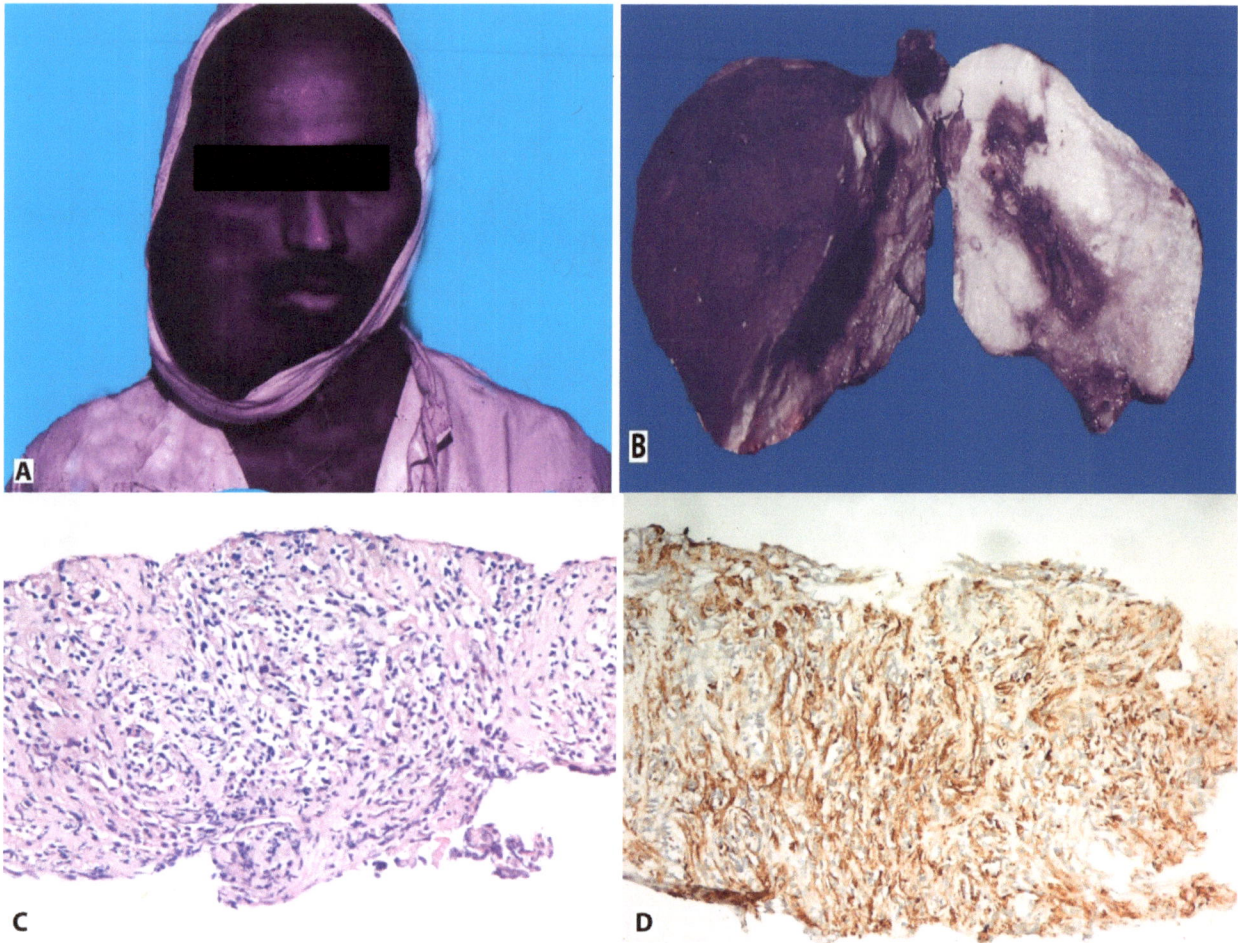

Figure 58 A case of leiomyosarcoma of cheek (A) a 30 year male presented with rapidly growing mass in lower half of right cheek, (B) widely resected mass of right cheek (C) spindle cell sarcoma (D) tumor cells express smooth muscle antigen

Myxoma

This is a mass of jelly like mucoid material with hypocellular myxoid change (Figure 59). It occurs typically in jaw bones and also within skeletal muscle belly anywhere. It behaves in a benign fashion.

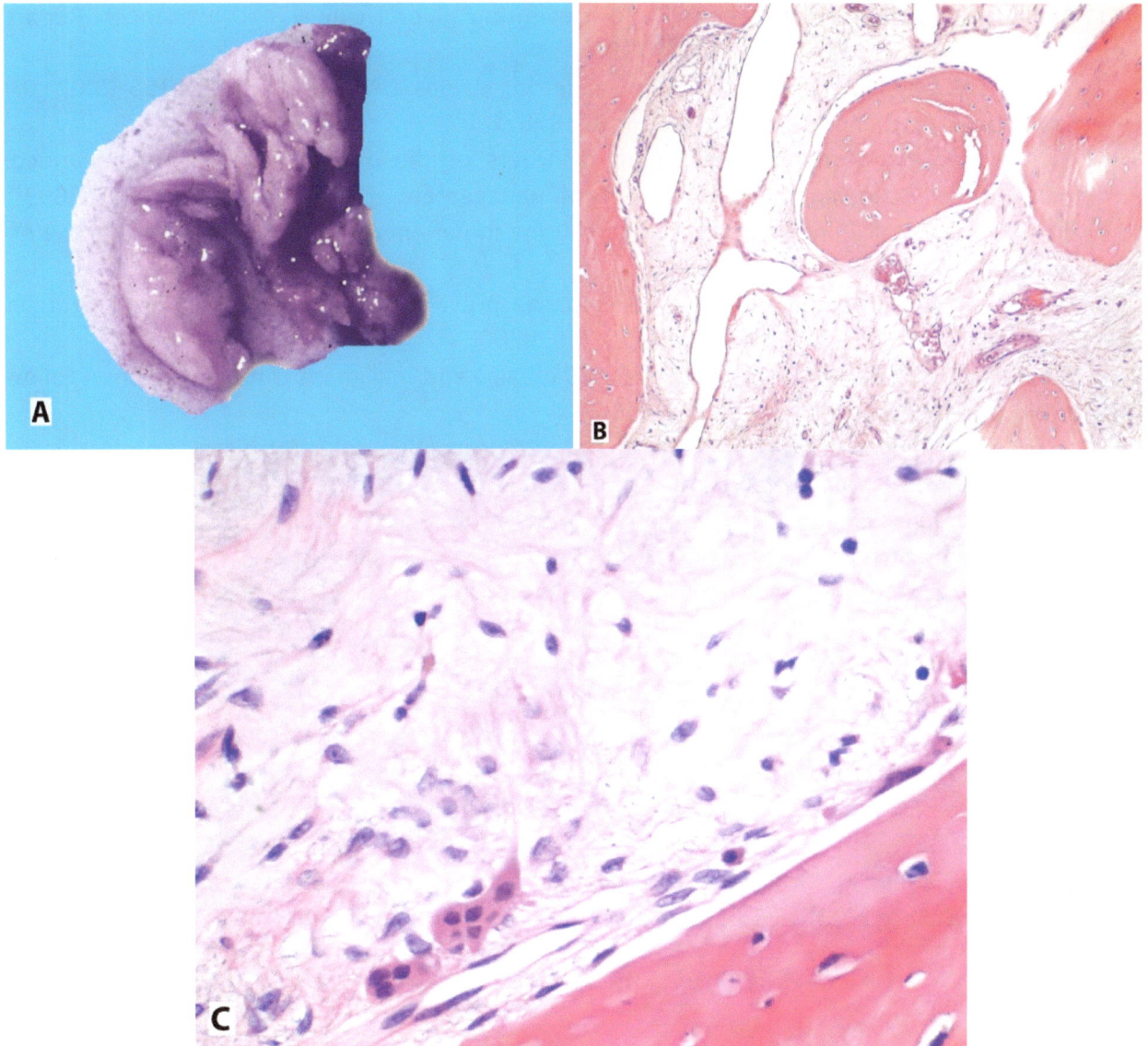

Figure 59 (A), Myxoma of mandible: white pink mucoid 2.5 cm mass enucleated from mandible, note a layer of whitish finely foamy mucin along left border, (B & C) typical myxoma relatively acellular and rich in edematous mucoid matrix

References:

Epithelial Precursor Lesions (premalignant lesions)

1) Axell T & Downer. Early diagnosis and prevention of oral cancer and precancer. Report on Symposium   AIII. Adv Dent Res. 9:134, 1995

2) Neville BW, Day TA. Oral cancer and precancerous lesions. CA Cancer J Clin 52:195, 2002

3) Kademani D Oral Cancer, Mayo Clin Proc 82: 878 ,2007

4) Waal I Van dor Potentially malignant disorders of the oral and oropharyngeal mucosa : terminology , classification and present concepts of management . Oral oncology 45 : 3 17, 2009

5) Einhorn J, Wersall J. Incidence of oral carcinoma in patients with leukoplakia of mucosa of the oral mucosa. Cancer 1967; 20:2189-219

5a) Petti S. Pooled estimate of world leukoplakia prevalence: a systematic review. Oral Oncol. 2003 Dec;39(8):770-80. Review. PubMed PMID: 13679200.

6) Silverman S Jr, Gorsky M, Lozada F. Oral leukoplakia and malignant transformation. A follow up study of 257 patient. Cancer 1984 ; 53:563-568

7) Wang Y P, Chen HM, Kuo RL ,etal . Oral verrucous Hyperplasia : histologic classification , prognosis , and clinical implications . J ozal Pathol Mod 38 : 651, 2009

8) Hosni ES Salum FG, Cherubini K , etal . Oral erythroplakia : retrospective analysis of 13 cases. Revista Brasileira de otozzinoloringologia. 75 :1, 2009

9) Fettig A, Pogrel in A , silverman S , etal . Proliferative verrucons leukoplakia of the gingival oral surg oral med oral pathol oral Radiol Endod 90 :723, 2000

10) ScullyC , Beyli M, Ferriro M, etal . update on oral Lichen Planus . Etiopathogenesis and Management . Crit Rev oral Biol Med 9 : 86 ,1998

11) Ismail SB, Kumar Sks Zain RB. Oral lichen Planus and lichenoid reactions. Etiopathogenesis , diagnosis management and malignant transformation J Oral Science 49 : 89 2007

12) Fatahzadeh M, Rinaggio J , Chido T squamous cell carcinoma arising in oral lichenoid lesion . JADA 135 :754, 2004

13) Angadi PV, Rekha KP. Oral submucous fibrosis: A clinic-pathologic review of 205 cases inIndia Oral Maxillofac Surg 2011; 15:15-19

Variants of Squamous cell Carcinoma of Oropharynx

14) Pereira MC , Oliveira DT , Landman G , Kowalski LP Histologic subtypes of oral squamous cell carcinoma J Can Dental Assoc 73 :339 ,2007

15) Stelow EB , Jo VY , stolar MH , Mills SE . Human Papilloma virus –associated squamous cell carcinoma of upper Aero- digestive Trant Am / Surg Pathol 34 :e15 2010

16) Badulescu Fl ,Crisan A, Badulescu A, Schenkar M. Recent data about the role of human papilloma virus (HPV in oncogenesis of head and neck cancer. Romanian Journal of morphology and embryology 51 : 437, 2010

17) Alkan A , Bulue E, Gunhano , Ozden B. Oral verrucous carcinoma Eur J Dent . 4: 202,2010

18) Fertilo A, Weiss LM, Rinaldo A, et al.Lymphoepithelial carcinoma of the larynx, hypopharynx and trachea. Ann Otol Rhinol Laryngol. 1997; 106:437-444

19) MacMillan C Kapadia SB, Finkelstein SD, et al. Lymphoepithelial carcinoma of the larynx and hypopharynx: study of 8 cases with relationship to Epstein-Barr virus p53 gene alterations, and review of the literature. Human Pathol 1996; 27:1172-1179

20) Choi HR Stargis Em , Rosenthal DI etal. Sarcomatoid carcinoma of head and neck , molecular Evidence for Evolution and Progression from conventional squamous cell carcinomas Am j Surg Pathol 27 : 1216, 2003

21) Weidner N. sarcomatoid carcinoma of the upper aerodigestive tract Semin Diagn Pathol 4: 157,1987

22) Gerughty RM, Henniger AR, Brown FM. Adenosquamous carcinoma of the nasal, oral and laryngeal cavities: A clinic-pathological survey of 10 cases. Cancer 1968; 22:1140-1155

23) Wieneke JA , Thompson LDR , Wenig BM .Basaloid squamous cell carcinoma of the sinonasal tract . Cancer 85 :841 ,1999

24) Ereno C, Gaafar A , Garmendia M etal. Basaloid squamous cell carcinoma of the head and neck . Head and Neck Pathol 2.83,2008

25) Banks ER Frierson HF mills 8E, etal . Basaloid squamous cell carcinoma of the Head and Neck . A clinicopathological and Immunohistochemical study of 40 cases Am j Surg Pathol 16 .939 ,1992

25a) Chernock RD, El-Mofty SK, Thorstad WL, Parvin CA, Lewis JS Jr. HPV-related nonkeratinizing squamous cell carcinoma of the oropharynx: utility of microscopic features in predicting patient outcome. Head Neck Pathol. 2009 Sep;3(3):186-94. doi: 10.1007/s12105-009-0126-1. Epub 2009 Jul 11. PubMed PMID: 20596971; PubMed Central PMCID: PMC2811624.

25b) Wain SL, Kier R, Vollmer RT, et al. Basaloid-squamous carcinoma of the tongue, hypopharynx and larynx: report of 10 cases. Hum Pathol. 1986;17(11):1158–66

26) Ferrer MJ Estelles E , Villanueva A, LopezR. Papillary squamous cell carcinoma of the oropharynx Euz Arch otorhinolaryngol 260 :444 ,2003

27) Jo Yv , Mills SE , stoler MH , Stelow EB. Papillary squamous cell carcinoma of the Head and Neck . Frequent Association with Human Papillomavirus Infection and Invasive carcinoma Am J Surg Pathol 33:1720,2009

28) Thompson LDR , Wenig BM, Hettner DK , Gnepp DR . Exophytic and papillary squamous cell carcinoma of the larynx : A clinicopathological series of 104 cases . Otolaryngol Head Neck Surg 1999; 120 :718

29) Folpe AL, Chand EM, Goldblum JR, Weiss SW. Expression of FLi-1, a nuclear transcription factor, distinguishes vascular neoplasms from mimics. Am J Surg Pathol 2001; 25:1061-1066

Lymphoproliferative Lesions of Head & Neck

Wegener's Granulomatosis

30) Hua F, Wilde B, Dolffs , Witzkeo T- lymphocytes and disease Mechanisms in Wegener's Granulomatosis . kidney Blood Press Res 32 :289 ,2009

31) Travis WD, Hoffman GS , Leavitt R ,etal Surgical Pathology of the Lung in Wegener's Granulomatosis . Review of 87 open lung Biopsies From 67 Patients Am J Surg Pathol 15 :315 ,1991

32) Devaney KO, Travis WD , Hoffman G , etal Interpretation of Head and Neck Biopies in Wegener ,s Granulomatosis . A Pathologic study of 126 Biopsies in 70 patients. Am J Surg Pathol 14 :555 ,1990

Nk/T cell Lymphoma

33) Watanable K, Hanamura A, Mori N. A unique caseof Nasal NK/T cell Lymphoma with Frequent Remission and Relapse showing Different Histological Features During 12 years of follow up .J Clin Exp Hematopathol 50 :65 ,2010

34) Li YX, Liu of Fang H et al. Variable clinical presentations of nasal and Waldeyer Ring natural Killer / T- cell Lymphoma . Clin cancer Res 15 : 2905 ,2009

35) Ko OB, Lee DH , Kim SW , etal . Clinicopathologic characteristics of T-cell Non Hodgkin lymphoma . A single Institution Experience Korean J Intern Med 24 :128 ,2009

36) Sitthinamsuwan P, Pongpruttipan T, Chularaojmontri L, et al. Extranodal NK/T cell lymphoma, nasal type, presenting with primary cutaneous lesion mimicking granuomatous panniculitis: a case report and review of literature 2010; 93:1001-1007

Sjogren's

37) Kass SS, GardyM. Sjorgen,s syndrome: an up date and overview. Am J Med; 1978; 64:1037-1046,

38) Pijpe J , Kalk WWl , Wal Je et al. Parotid gland biopsy compared with labial biopsy in the diagnosis of patients with Primary Sjogren's Syndrome. Rheumatology 43 : 335 , 2007

39) Zulman J, Jaffe R, Talat N. Evidence that the malignant lymhom of Sjogren's síndrome is a monoclonal B cell lymphoma. N Engl J Med 1978; 299, 1215-1220

Lymphomatoid Granulomatosis

40) Makol A, Kosuri K, Tamkas D etal. Lymphomatoid Granulomatosis masquerading as interstitial pneumonia in a 66-year old man : a case report and review of literature . J Hematol & Oncol,2009; 2 : 39

41) Katzenstein A-LA, Carrington CB, Liebow AA. Lymphomatoid granulomatosis: A clinico-pathologic study of 152 cases. Cancer 1979; 43:360-373

42) Liebow AA, Carrington CRB, Frieman PJ. Lymphomatoid granulomatosis Hum Pathol 1972; 3:457-558

42a): Magro CM, Dyrsen M. Angiocentric lesions of the head and neck. Head Neck Pathol. 2008 Jun;2(2):116-30. doi: 10.1007/s12105-008-0049-2. Epub 2008 May 27. PubMed PMID: 20614334; PubMed Central PMCID: PMC2807549

Carcinomas of Sino-nasal Tract & Salivary Glands

43) Hickman RE, Cawson RA, Duffy SW. The Prognosis of Specific Type of Salivary Gland Tumors Cancer 1984; 54:1620-1624

43a) Ejaz A, Wenig BM. Sinonasal undifferentiated carcinoma: clinical and pathologic features and a discussion on classification, cellular differentiation and differential diagnosis. Adv Anat Pathol. 2005 May;12(3):134-43. Review. PubMed PMID: 15900114.

43b). Frierson HF Jr, Mills SE, Fechner RE, et al. Sinonasal undifferentiated carcinoma. An aggressive neoplasm derived from Schneiderian epithelium and distinct from olfactory neuroblastoma Am J Surg Pathol. 1986; 10:771–779.

44) Ritland F, Lubensky I, LiVolsy VA. Polymorphous low-grade-adenocarcinoma of the parotid salivary gland. Arch Pathol Lab Med 1993; 117:1261-1263

45) Lewis JE, McKinney BC, Weiland LH, et al. Salivary duct carcinoma. Clinico-pathologic and immunohistochemical review of 26 cases Cancer 1996; 77:223-230

46) Seethala RR, Hunt JL, Baloch ZW, et al. Adenoid cystic carcinoma with high-grade transformation: a report of 11 cases and a review of the literature 2007; 31:1683-1694

47) Savera AT, sloman A, Huvos AG, Klimstra DS. Myoepithelial carcinoma of the salivary glands A clinicopathological study of 25 patients Am J Surg Pathol 2000; 24:761-774

48) Nagao T, Sugan I , Ishida Y, etal. Hybrid carcinoma of the salivary glands : report of nine cases with clinic-pathologic Immunohistochemical, and P53 gene Alteration Analysis Mod Pathol 2002; 15 :724-733

49) Seethal RR , Barnes EL , Hunt JL Epithelial –Myoepithelial carcinoma : A review of the clinico pathological spectrums and immunophenotypic characteristics in 61 tumor of the salivary glands and upper Aero- digestive Am J Surg Pathol 31 :44,2007

50) Cho kj, el-Naggar AK, Ordonez NG, et al Epithelial-myoepithelial carcinoma of salivary glands; A clinicopathologic. DNA flow cytometry, and immunohistochemical study of Ki67 and Her 2/neu oncogene Am J Clin Pathol 1995;l 103:432-437

Malignant Mixed Tumor (Carcinosarcoma)

51) Fowler MH , Fowler J Ducatman B , et al. Malignant mixed tumors of the Salivary glands: a study of loss of heterozygosity in tumor suppressor genes Mod Pathol 19 :350 ,2006

52) Horky JK, Chaloupka JC , Putman CM , etal . True malignant mixed Tumor (Carcinosarcoma) of Tonsillar Minor Salivary gland origin: Diagnostic imaging and Endovascular Therapeutic Embolization AJNR 18: 1944,1997

53) Gnepp DR. Malignant Mixed Tumors of the Salivary Gland Pathol Annu1993; 28 (part 1): 279:328

54) Antoni J, Gopalan V, Smith RA, et al. Carcinoma ex pleomorphic adenoma: a comprehensive review of clinical, pathological and molecula4 data Head & Neck 2012; 6:1-9

55) Lewis JE, Olsen KD, Sebo TJ. Carcinoma ex pleomorphic adenoma: pathologic analysis of 73 cases Hum Pathol 2001; 32:5960604

56) Czader M, Eberhart EB, Bhatti N, et al. Metastasizing Mixed Tumor of the Parotid: Initial presentation as a solitary kidney tumor and ultimate carcinomatous transformation at the prior site Am J Surg Pathol 2000; 24;1159-1164

Melanotic Neuroectodermal Tumor Of Infancy

57) George JC, Edwards MK, Jakacki RI Kho –Duffin J . Melanotic Neuroecto dermal Tumor of Infancy AJNR AMJ Neuroradiol 1995; 16:1273 -1275

58) Patankar T, Prasad , Goels , etal. Malignant melanotic neuroectodermal Tumor of Infancy affecting the occipital squama J Postgrd Med 1998; 44:73 -75

Olfactory Neuroblastoma

59) Lewis JS Jr. Ferlito A, Gnepp DR, et al. Terminology and classification of neuroendocrine neoplasms of the larynx. Laryngoscope. 2011;121:1187–1193.

59a) Sorensen PH , WUJK Berean Kuv , etal. Olfactory Neuroblastoma is a peripheral primitive neuroectodermal tumor related to Ewing's sarcoma Proc Natl Acad Sci USA 1996; 93:1038-1043

60) Thompson LDR olfactory Neuroblastoma. Head and Neck Pathol 2009; 3 :252 -259

61) KOO BK, AN JH , JEON KH , etal .Two cases of Ectopic Adrenocorticotrophic Hormone syndrome with olfactory Neuroblastoma and Literature Review. Endocrine Journal 2008; 55:469-475

62) Josephs L Jones L, Marenette L, Mckeever P . Cushings syndrome An Unusual Presentation of olfactory Neuroblastoma Skull Base 2008; 18: 73 -76

63) Vranic s , caughron SK, Djuricic S etal . Hamartomas, teratomas and teratocarcinomas of the head and neck . Report of 3 cases with clinico-pathological correlation cytogenetic analysis and review of the literature Ear , Nose and throat Disorders . BMC 5; 8: 2008

Mucosal Malignant Melanoma Of Head & Neck

64) Alfred E. Chang, M.D. Lucy Hynds Karnell, Ph.D, Herman R. Menck, M.B.A .Report on Cutaneous and Noncutaneous Melanoma: A Summary of 84,836 Cases from the Past Decade
Cancer 1998; 83; 1664-1678

65) Thompson LDR , Wieneke/ JA , Miettinen M. Sinonasal tract and Nasopharyngeal melanomas : A clinicopathological study of 115 cases with a proposed staging system Am J Surg Pathol 2003; 27 :594-611

66) Prasad ML, Jungbluth AA, Iverson K , etal. Expression of melanocytic Differentiation markers in malignant melanomas of the oral and sinonasal mucosa Am J Surg Pathol 25:782, 2001

67) Prasad ML, Patel S, Hoshaw –Woodward S ,et al. Prognostic Factors for malignant melanoma of the squamous mucosa of the head & neck Am J Surg Pathol 2002; 26 :883-892

Paragangliomas

68) Alford BR, Guilford FR. A comprehensive study of tumors of the glomus jugulare Laryngoscope72:765, 1962

69) Johnstone PAS, Foss RD, Desilets DJ. Malignant Jugulo-tympanic paraganglioma Arch Pathol Lab Med. 114:975

70) Levit SA, Sheps SG, Espinosa RE, et al. Catecholamine-secreting paraganglioma of the glomus jugulare region resembling pheochromocytoma. N Engl J Med 281:805, 1969

71) Tannir NM, Cortas N, Allam C. A functioning catecholamine-secreting vagal body tumor: A case report and review of the literature. Cancer 52: 932, 1983

72) Green JD, Olsen KD, DeSanto LW, Scheithauer BW. Neoplasms of vagus nerve. Laryngoscope98:648, 1988

73) Heinrich MC, Harris AE, Bell WR. Metastatic intravagale paraganglioma: Case report and review of the literature. Am J Med 78:1017, 1985

74) Arias-Stella J, Valcarcel J. Chief cell hyperplasia in human carotid body at high altitude. Physiological and pathological significance. Hum Pathol 7:361

75) Lack EE. Hyperplasia of vagal and carotid body paraganglia in patients with chronic hypoxemia.am J Pathol 91:497, 1978

76) Rodriguez-Cuevas H, Lopez-Garza J, Labstida-Almendara S. Carotid body tumors in inhabitants of altitudes higher than 2000 meters above sea levek. Head Neck 20:374, 1998

77) Sajid MS, Hamilton G, Baker M. A multicentric review of carotid body tumor management. Eur J Vasc Endovasc Surg 34:127, 2007

78) Lack EE, Cubilla AL, Woodruff JM. Paragangliomas of head and neck region: A clinical study of 69 patients. Cancer 39: 397, 1977

79) Lack EE, Cubilla AL, Woodruff JM. Paragangliomas of the head and neck region: A pathological study of tumors from 71 patients. Hum Pathol 10:191, 1979

80) Gruferman S, Gillman MW, Pasternak LR, et al. Familial carotid body tumors: Case report and epidemiological review. Cancer 46:2116, 1980

81) Zbareb P, Lehmann W. Carotid body Paraganglioma with Metastases. Laryngoscope 95:450, 1985

82) Lee JH, Barich F, Karnell LH, et al. National Cancer data report on malignant paragangliomas of the head and neck. Cancer 94:730, 2002

83) Ferlito A, Barnes L, Wenig BM. Identification, classification, treatment and prognosis of laryngeal paraganglioma. Review of the literature and eight new cases. Ann Otol Rhinol Laryngol 103:525, 1994

84) Maisel R, Schmidt D, Pambuccian S Subglottic laryngeal paraganglioma. Laryngoscope 113:401, 2003

85) Myssiorek D, Rinaldo A. Barnes L, Ferlito A. Laryngeal paraganglioma: an updated critical review. Acta Laryngol. 124:995, 2004

86) Lack EE, Stillinger RA, Colvin DB et al. Aortico-Pulmonary paraganglioma: report of a case with ultrastructural study and review of literature. Cancer 43:269, 1979

87) Johnson TL, Lloyd RV, Shapiro B, et al. Cardiac paragangliomas: a clinico-pathological and immunohistochemical study of four cases. Am J Surg Pathol 1985; 9:827

88) Lack EE. Aortico-Pulmonary Paragangliomas and Paragangliomas of the Lung, in Pathology of Adrenal and Extra-Adrenal Paragangliomas, Major Problems in Pathology Vol 29 W B Saunders, Philadelphia, 1994

89) Olson JL, Salyer WR. Mediastinal paragangliomas (aortic body tumor): a report of 4 cases and review of the literature. Cancer 1978; 41:2405,

90) Pellitteri PK, Rinaldo A, Myssiorek D, et al. Paragangliomas of the head and neck Oral Oncol. 2004; 40:563,

Mesenchymal Tumors of Head & Neck

91) Fletcher CDM. Distinctive Soft Tissues Tumors of the Head & Neck. Mod Pathol 2002; 15:324-330

92) Bremer JW, Neel HB, DeSanto LW, et al. Angiofibroma: treatment trends in 150 patients during 40 years. Laryngoscope 1986; 96:1321-1329

93) Herman P, LOT G, Chapot R, et al. Long term follow up of juvenile nasopharyngeal angiofibromas: analysis of recurrences. Laryngoscope 1999; 109:140-147

94) Hwang HC, Mills SE, Patterson K, et al. Expression of androgen receptors in nasopharyngeal angiofibroma; an immunohistochemical study of 24 cases. Mod Pathol 1998; 11:1122-1106

95) Thompson LDR, Miettinen M Wenig BM. Sino-nasal type Hemangiopericytoma: A clinicopathological and immunophenotypic Analysis of 104 Cases Showing Perivascular Myoid Differentiation Am J Surg Pathol 2003; 27:737-749

www.ingramcontent.com/pod-product-compliance
Lightning Source LLC
Chambersburg PA
CBHW041702200326

41518CB00002B/160